COMPREHENSIVE GUIDE TO UNDERSTANDING AND TREATING ACNE-PRONE SKIN

AN IN-DEPTH OVERVIEW OF INGREDIENTS, TREATMENTS & PREVENTION

KARINA THOMAS

COMPREHENSIVE GUIDE TO UNDERSTANDING AND TREATING ACNE-PRONE SKIN

TABLE OF CONTENTS

INTRODUCTION

In the field of skin care and dermatology, not many conditions are as widely researched and documented as acne. Acne is a skin condition that can affect people of all ages, from infants to adults. It is characterized by the appearance of pimples, blackheads, whiteheads, and/or cysts on the skin. While it is most commonly seen on the face, it can also appear on other parts of the body, such as the chest, back, and shoulders.

The scientific body and research on the subject have been growing exponentially in recent years, with new findings and treatments being discovered all the time. Acne is now better understood than ever before, and there are a number of effective treatments available for those who suffer from it.

However, despite all of this progress, there is still a lot of misinformation out there about acne and its treatment. This can make it difficult for people to know what to believe, and how to find the information they need to make informed decisions about their skincare.

We begin the guide by going into detail about acne, what it is, its causes, and how to identify it. We will then move on to discuss the various treatments that are available for acne, both medical and natural.

We'll delve deeper into some of the most effective ingredients used in acne treatments, both over-the-counter and prescription. And we'll also provide some tips on how to choose the right product for your clients, based on their individual needs.

This guide is designed to be a comprehensive resource for anyone who is looking to learn more about acne and its treatment. Whether you're a skincare professional or someone who suffers from the condition, we hope you'll find the information here helpful and informative.

So without further ado, let's get started.

CHAPTER 1:
UNDERSTANDING THE BASICS OF ACNE

In order to understand the top and other conditions of the skin, it is essential to have a great understanding of skin structure and function. This chapter centers on the basic physiology and anatomy of the skin.

The skin is an astounding organ that's essential for life. One cannot live without skin. It performs numerous crucial capacities that offer assistance to many other functions of the body. Our skin reacts to hormones, biochemicals, and signals sent from numerous other organs and tissues within the body. It is the first line of defense against malady and outside intruders attempting to enter the body.

When we think about our body organs, we might think about the heart or the liver or maybe the brain, but the skin is the biggest organ within the body. An average size person's skin weighs around 8 pounds or 15 percent of a person's body weight, and in case you extended all the skin out from the average person's body, it would take up almost 18 square feet. The skin is a complicated covering that makes a difference in cushioning and protecting the rest of the body.

The primary functions of the skin are to protect the body from infection and injury, regulate body temperature, and excrete waste products. The skin helps to protect the body from infection by acting as a barrier to bacteria, viruses, and other harmful organisms.

Layers of Skin

The skin is made up of three principal layers which are:

- ➢ **Epidermis**
- ➢ **Dermis**
- ➢ **Subcutaneous Tissue**

The epidermis is the farthest layer of skin that you just see. It's also the most slender layer of skin, averaging only 0.5 mm in thickness. The main function of the epidermis is to protect the body from infection and injury.

The epidermis is further divided into four sublayers. ***The stratum corneum, stratum lucidum, stratum granulosum, and stratum spinosum***. The stratum corneum is the outermost layer of the epidermis. It's also the layer that you see when you look in the mirror. This layer is made up of dead skin cells that are held together by a protein called keratin. The stratum corneum acts as a barrier to protect the body from infection and injury.

The stratum Lucidum is the second layer of the epidermis. This layer is made up of living skin cells that are filled with keratin. The stratum granulosum is the third layer of the epidermis which consists of dead skin cells that are filled with protein. The stratum spinosum is the fourth layer of the epidermis. This fourth layer comprises living skin cells that are connected to each other by tiny fibers called desmosomes.

The dermis is the middle layer of skin that contains blood vessels, sweat glands, hair follicles, and other structures. This layer is much thicker than the epidermis, averaging 2 mm in thickness.

The dermis is further divided into two sublayers. The ***papillary region*** and the ***reticular region***. The papillary region is the upper layer of the dermis. This layer is made up of thin, finger-like projections called papillae. The papillae are connected to the epidermis by a network of tiny blood vessels called capillaries. The reticular region is the lower layer of the dermis which is made up of thick, interwoven fibers that provide strength and support to the skin.

The subcutaneous tissue is the innermost layer of skin that consists of fat and connective tissue. This layer helps to keep the skin attached to the underlying muscles and bones. The subcutaneous tissue has further two sublayers. The ***hypodermis*** and the ***dermis***. The hypodermis is the innermost layer of the subcutaneous tissue. The hypodermis is the layer of fat and connective tissue that is located beneath the skin and connective tissue that helps to cushion and protect the body.

Skin and Immune System

The skin and the immune system work together to protect the body from infection and disease. The skin provides a physical barrier that prevents harmful microorganisms from entering the body. The immune cells in the skin help to identify and destroy harmful microbes.

The antimicrobial peptides that are produced by the skin help to inhibit the production of harmful microorganisms. The beneficial microorganisms that live on the skin benefit the body from damage.

The skin also contains a variety of antimicrobial peptides; these peptides are produced by the skin cells in response to infection or injury, which produce substances that would be hurtful to intruders.

The immune system comprises specialized cells within the blood as well as in the skin. One of the most important resistant cells is the Langerhans cell, which wanders through the mid-epidermis and dermis. The Langerhan cell function is to identify the outside bodies within the skin and to signal biochemical reactions that cause the skin and immune system to respond against foreign bodies.

White blood cells are also important in acne because they help to fight infection and inflammation. The white blood cells that are most effective in fighting acne are neutrophils, macrophages, and lymphocytes. Lymphocytes are white blood cells that help to regulate the immune system.

The Pathophysiology of Acne

Acne cannot be defined more simply than a blockage of oil and dead cells in the pores of our skin, mostly on facial areas. These pores are commonly known as hair holes which get blocked for many reasons which will be discussed later.

Acne is a condition of the skin that occurs when the hair follicles got to be blocked with oil and dead skin cells from the sebum. The blockage causes the sebaceous glands to become inflamed and enlarged, which can lead to pimples, blackheads, and whiteheads.

The anatomy of the hair follicle and sebaceous gland are essential to understanding how acne develops. The hair follicle is a small tube that extends from the surface of the skin down to the subcutaneous layer. The sebaceous gland is attached to the hair follicle and produces sebum, an oily substance that lubricates and waterproofs the skin.

Sebum is produced by the sebaceous glands and is composed of triglycerides, wax esters, and squalene. When the sebaceous glands produce too much sebum, it can combine with dead skin cells and block the hair follicles. This blockage can cause the follicles to become inflamed and enlarged, which leads to the development of pimples, blackheads, and whiteheads.

The 4 Factors Involved In Development

Four internal factors that might contribute to acne development are:

1. **High sebum production** - During adolescence when androgen, a male sex hormone, is produced at high levels. This overproduction of androgen stimulates the sebaceous glands to produce more sebum. Sebum production can also be increased by certain medications, such as corticosteroids, androgens, and lithium.

2. **Hyperkeratinization** - The process of keratinization is the conversion of keratinocytes, the cells that make up the majority of the epidermis, into keratin. Hyperkeratinization occurs when there is an overproduction of keratinocytes. This overproduction can be ascribed to a bunch of factors, including hormonal changes, medications, and certain skin conditions. When hyperkeratinization occurs, the excess keratinocytes can block the hair follicles and cause the development of pimples, blackheads, and whiteheads.

3. **Cutibacterium acnes** - Cutibacterium acnes (also commonly known as *Propionibacterium acnes*) is a bacteria that lives on the skin. This bacteria feeds on sebum and can cause the follicles to

become blocked. When the follicles are blocked, C. acnes can grow and multiply, which can trigger acne to occur.

4. **Hormonal Changes** - Hormonal changes, such as those that occur during puberty, menstruation, and pregnancy, can also contribute to the development of acne. These changes play a vital role in acne production and severity which will be discussed in detail further.

Acne may develop on any part of the body but we mostly find them on our face, neck, back, and shoulders. With acne, we might see discoloration of the skin with some roughness as well. The most common type of acne is called acne vulgaris, which involves the inflammation of the hair follicles.

So till now in this chapter, we have discussed the physiology of the skin, layers of skin, and how skin and immunity are related. Conjointly, we have discussed how acne develops in the skin. The types and causes of acne will be discussed in the following chapters.

CHAPTER 2
BIOLOGY OF ACNE

This chapter includes the biological definition of acne along with processes, and how we can relate acne with genetics and heredity. Before going towards definition, let us have a view of the fact that acne is much more common than any other skin disease. So whatever information will be shared in this chapter must not be shocking for readers as almost every one of us have to deal with acne at some point of time in our lives.

Biological Definition of Acne

"Acne is an inflammatory disorder of the skin, which has sebaceous (oil) glands that connect to the hair follicle, which contains fine hair."

Cell Renewal in the Follicle

Every day, our skin cells are subjected to damage from UV rays, pollution, and other environmental stressors. This damage can cause the cells to become damaged or unhealthy. In order to maintain healthy skin, our body must constantly renew the skin cells. The process of cell renewal is known as cell turnover.

The cells in the uppermost layer of our skin, the epidermis, are constantly shedding and being replaced by new cells. Our skin normally sheds dead skin through a process called "desquamation". The new and modern cells are produced in the most profound layer of the epidermis which is the stratum germinativum.

The cells in the stratum germinativum continue to divide and produce new cells. These new cells move up through the layers of the skin and eventually reach the surface. As they travel, the cells change shape and form, becoming flat and scale-like. The process of cell turnover takes about 28 days from start to finish its process in the entire body.

Once the dead skin cells are discarded they get settled on the ground or furniture which means that many of the times the dust in your home is not dirt only but, rather, dead skin cells.

This cell renewal process does not work proficiently in people with acne because this natural desquamation process in them gets lost. Those people with acne-prone skins are more likely to have a condition called *retention hyperkeratosis* in which dead skins are produced more than typical and are not properly shed.

How Speeding Up Turnover Results

The rate at which our cells turn over slows down as we age which is the reason why our skin starts to look flaky as we grow old. The rate of turnover is twice as fast as adults which always makes their skin look smooth and bright.

Individuals with acne-prone skins need to fasten up the process of turnover by outside means. This is why it is important to use products that encourage cell turnovers, such as exfoliants and retinoids. Exfoliants help to remove the dead skin cells that can build up on the surface of the skin and clog pores. Retinoids help to speed up the cell turnover process, which can help to reduce the appearance of wrinkles and fine lines.

Presentation of Acne

There are multiple ways in which acne can form. Pimples, scarring, and inflammation, for example, are three of the most common forms of acne. Firstly, it is essential to understand not to mix or confuse these forms with acne types, they will be explained in a later section.

> ➢ **Pimples** - A pimple is the most commonly occurring form of acne, which is also known as a papule (type of acne). A pimple is a small, raised bump on the surface of the skin that can be red, white, or yellow in color. Pimples are typically filled with pus and can be painful to the touch.

> ➢ **Inflammation** - Inflammation is the most painful form of acne, which is also known as erythema. Inflammation appears as a red, swollen area on the surface of the skin that can result in constant pain. Inflammation typically occurs when the C. acne bacteria develop, they emit squander products and enzymes. These harm skin cells and trigger an immune reaction coming about in aroused acne.

> ➢ **Scarring** - Scarring is the third most common form of acne, also known as atrophic scarring. Scarring is a permanent change to the texture of the skin that can be raised or sunken in appearance. Depending on its intensity, acne can cause emotional distress and scarring. People often do popping up their pimples which increases the ratio of scarring. So one must not go for popping no matter how tempting or easy it may look, it would not result in a better way.

Genetics and Heredity

Simply put, if your parents had acne, you are at higher risk to have it as well. In fact, studies have shown that up to 80% of people with acne have a family history of the condition. Acne can run in families, but many people with acne do not have affected people in their families. It is likely that a combination of genetic, hormonal, and lifestyle factors (such as diet, stress, skincare products, etc) act in combination to cause most acne.

The study, published in Nature Communications, looked at the DNA of 26,722 people, including 5,602 who have severe acne. Researchers identified genetic variations in 15 genome regions that were more common in people with severe acne.

Different Skin Types

In dermatology, skin type is defined as the level of skin pigmentation in the skin. These skin pigmentation levels are associated with the origin of race and ethnicity. All of the ethnic pigmentation levels are linked genetically.

According to research, a universal scale Fitzpatrick Skin Typing is used to examine the skin pigmentation levels in the person's skin and also to calculate any individual resistant capacity to sunburn and sun exposure damage.

The different skin types range from Type I to Type IV, lightest skin color for Type I, and darkest skin color for Type IV. To understand the variation in acne due to differences let us understand each type first.

Type I - The Fitzpatrick skin type I is the lightest skin color and it is associated with people of Northern European descent. The people with this skin type are very fair, have blonde or red hair, and blue or green eyes. They always burn in the sun and never tan.

Type II - The Fitzpatrick skin type II is also light skin color, but it is not as light as Type I. This skin type is linked with people of Southern European descent. Individuals with this skin type are fair, have blonde or red hair, and blue or green eyes. They sometimes burn in the sun and sometimes tan.

Type III - The Fitzpatrick skin type III is medium skin color and it is affiliated with people of Mediterranean, Middle Eastern, or Hispanic descent. Those people who have this type of skin are olive, have dark hair, and have brown eyes. They occasionally burn in the sun and always tan.

Type IV - The Fitzpatrick skin type IV is dark skin color and it is connected with people of African, Asian, or Hispanic descent. The people with this skin type are brown, have black hair, and have brown eyes. Those people almost never burn in the sun and always tan.

Esthetic Skin Typing

In esthetics, skin type alludes to the oiliness level of the skin and how much sebum is produced in particular zones of the face. Esthetic skin types are measured by the size and dispersion of obvious pores on the skin, which links specifically to the oiliness level of the skin. This level of oiliness and dryness of any individual has genetic reasons because our genes decide the production level and size of sebaceous glands in almost every part of the skin. Pore size is additionally genetic. When sebum is produced by the sebaceous glands, it creates stretching in the walls of follicles, causing the appearance of enlarged pores.

A large UK study involving 400 twin pairs showed that 81% of acne was due to hereditary factors. Research about genetic factors of acne has shown that there is no single gene that is responsible for causing acne. Rather, it seems to be a combination of several different genes that can contribute to the development of acne.

This chapter enlightened that acne is a complex condition that is influenced by both genetic and lifestyle factors. While there is no single cure for acne, understanding the various contributing factors can help to develop an effective treatment plan. In addition, knowing your skin type can be helpful in choosing the right skincare products and avoiding potential triggers. For the treatment and best skin care products look forward to our following chapters.

CHAPTER 3
TYPES AND CAUSES OF ACNE

Acne has several kinds including fungal acne. But most of the time people find themselves having simple acne with blockage of oil and dead cells. We normally call them whiteheads, blackheads, and pimples. These are visible types of acne, though very small in a size other types are mostly not visible to the naked human eye. These blockages in pores are also known as comedones. They can be open and close-ended. As the size of any comedone increases, it results in the rupture of the wall of the hair follicle. This happening is the root cause of redness, inflammation, and itching on the skin. If the blockage in pores is deepened it may develop irritation, pain, and puss as well.

Types of Acne

There are four types of acne that dermatologists and skin specialists normally identify. These types include:

1. Comedonal acne

2. Papular

3. Pustular

4. Nodular

Comedonal Acne

Comedonal acne is the most common type of acne and is characterized by blackheads and whiteheads. If you have comedonal acne it might take 8 weeks to notice an improvement. Comedones are considered non-inflammatory acne lesions that may be open and closed. A single lesion is a comedo. Comedonal acne appears in six forms:

> ➤ *Open comedones* are blackheads; the black color is because of the surface pigment (melanin).

> ➤ *Closed comedones* are whiteheads; that occur when the follicle gets completely blocked.

> ➤ *Microcomedones*; they are so small in size that can not be visible to the naked eye.

> ➤ *Macrocomedones* are facial blocked comedones that are bigger than 2mm in diameter.

> ➤ *A giant comedo*; is a big, black-colored bump that is greater than 5mm in diameter. It is a type of cyst.

> ➤ *Solar comedo*; is caused by sun damage and excessive exposure to ultraviolet radiation. They are seen on the chin and cheeks of older people.

Blackheads

These are open bumps on the skin that fill with an overabundance of oil and dead skin. It looks like the dirt has been stored within the bump, but the dull sports are really caused by sporadic light reflection off the clogged follicle.

Typically when a "plug" made up of oil and dead skin cells gets stuck in the opening of a hair follicle. This plug oxidizes and turns black, hence they get named "blackheads."

The blackhead usually occurs on the tip of the nose but can also be spotted on the chest, back, shoulders, and arms. Because of their dark color, blackheads are simple to spot on the skin. They are marginally raised, in spite of the fact that they are not painful since they are not aroused like pimples.

Whiteheads

When the plugged follicle is closed off by a covering of skin, it shows up white. Usually called a whitehead and is competent at remaining within the skin for a long time. It may moreover end up aroused or advance into another frame. These are relatively firm and can not be pressed empty since the comedo is not in communication with the skin surface.

Whiteheads are similar to blackheads, but they're usually smaller and have a white or yellowish appearance. However, numerous grown-ups proceed to have whiteheads into their 20s, 30s, and beyond. A few indeed develop whiteheads for the very first time as adults. Like blackheads, whiteheads are also likely to appear on your face, back, and neck. In very rare cases they can also develop on your hips, thighs, and armpits. Whiteheads generally go away on their own, but it may take a small time, maybe up to 7 days.

Papular Acne

Papular acne is characterized by small, raised bumps that are not filled with pus. Papules are small, raised bumps that can appear on the surface of the skin. They're often red or pink and can be tender to the touch. Papules are a type of inflammatory acne, meaning they develop when the hair follicle becomes inflamed or irritated. Papules do not have a yellow or white center of pus. When a papule does gather pus, it gets to be a postulate.

In case the comedone breaks and scatters the microbes into the skin tissues, as contradicted on the skin surface, your body will react with irritation to fight the microbes. This aroused lesion may be a papule. Moreover, if you have a papule that's huge and appears to be particularly swollen and excruciating, it might not actually be a papule. It can be an acne nodule.

Pustular Acne

Pustular acne causes large, raised bumps that are filled with pus. Pus is a yellowish or white fluid that's made up of dead skin cells, oil, and bacteria. Acne pustules show up differently from the other types of acne imperfections. Pustules tend to happen close to oil glands, particularly around the face, back, and shoulders.

They can shift in measure from exceptionally little to very expansive. Pustules are also a type of inflammatory acne. White blood cells assemble on the papule to fight against the contamination as the pore breaks down. These cells form the pus you see inside the blemish. They seem like whiteheads encompassed by red rings. They can cause scarring in case they are picked or scratched.

Nodular Acne

Nodular acne is the most severe type of acne which includes cysts and nodules. If the clogged pores are deeper and more irritated, they can even turn into painful, deep nodules - solid lumps - and cysts - pus-filled lumps. Nodular acne may also be skin toned. Nodules may continue for weeks or indeed months, with the result of their substance hardening into profound and may be persistent cysts.

Nodular and cystic acne are the worst kinds and tend to leave the deepest scars. Both cysts and nodules can be painful and may last for weeks or months if they're not treated.

Subtypes of Acne

Acne has many subtypes as well. ***Acne neonatorum*** and ***Acne infantum*** occasionally affect newborns and infants, usually boys. A pimply rash appears on the face and usually clears within weeks with no lasting effect. However, acne infantum may last longer, be more severe, and cause scarring. People who escaped their teen years almost pimple-free may develop persistent adult-onset acne as they get older.

Despite the normal increase in androgen levels during puberty, some doctors believe that flare-ups of acne have less to do with androgen levels than with how a person's skin responds to an increase in sebum production or to the bacteria that causes acne. The bacteria Propionibacterium acnes occur naturally in healthy hair follicles.

If too many of them accumulate in plugged follicles, they may secrete enzymes that break down sebum and cause inflammation. Some people are simply more sensitive than others to this reaction. Sebum levels that might cause a pimple or two in one person may result in widespread outbreaks.

Causes of Acne

Acne is not a disease bracketed to any age but it is most common among teenagers, especially with a bit of an unhealthy lifestyle, but it can affect people of all ages. Doctors still don't know exactly why some people experience acne and others don't, although almost 90% of people have acne at some point of time in their lives.

According to a systematic analysis for the Global Burden of Disease Study, in 2010, the prevalence of acne among the population in the world was 9.38%, ranking eighth in the world.

There are countless reasons for acne, but the prime cause is still a mystery. However, experts have possible explanations for acne development. Following are some of the causes:

Certain Medications

Acne can be a side effect of certain medications, such as corticosteroids, testosterone, lithium, some types of hormonal birth control, anticonvulsants, and steroids family history of acne. If you think your medication is causing acne, talk to your doctor about other options

Hormonal Imbalance

You may have noticed that you seem to break out more during stressful times in your life. This is not random! Our hormones are greatly impacted by stress, which has an impact on the skin. Our endocrine system secretes more cortisol when we are stressed out. The body will prioritize the production of cortisol over sex hormones during prolonged periods of stress. This frequently results in decreased progesterone, which can contribute to breakouts. Additionally, cortisol can cause insulin spikes, which in turn cause more androgen (testosterone) production, which in turn causes more acne.

One has the highest risk of developing acne during puberty. During that time, your body undergoes many hormonal changes. These changes can trigger oil production, leading to an increased risk of acne. Hormonal acne related to puberty usually improves when you reach adulthood, and your breakouts may even stop completely. Other hormonal imbalances can also cause acne. These include polycystic ovary syndrome (PCOS), pregnancy, and menopause.

Air Pollution

Our most prevalent skin conditions are becoming more and more linked to air pollution. Air pollution has been shown to affect psoriasis, acne, hyperpigmentation, atopic dermatitis, and other skin conditions. It is essential to include pollution as a risk factor for these skin conditions; consequently, we must discuss ways to mitigate its negative effects with patients. Any chemical, physical, or biological agent that alters the natural characteristics of the atmosphere is considered to be air pollution when it affects both the outdoor (ambient) and indoor (household) environments.

In one study, people who lived in areas with high levels of air pollution were more facing problems with acne. It is the most challenging natural issue for almost every country, especially in Chinese cities.

Clinical studies reported that air pollutants had a deleterious effect on the skin by increasing oxidative stress, leading to a severe change in the normal functions of lipids, deoxyribonucleic acid, and/or proteins in the human skin.

Psychological Factors

Psychological factors actuate the discharge of neuropeptides and hormones that activate cells to take interest in acne issues. If you have acne, you may be more likely to have anxiety and depression as well. Some research shows that people who have acne tend to have higher levels of the stress hormone cortisol. Cortisol signals your body to make more oil which results in acne.

Temperature And Humidity

Changes in temperature and humidity can make acne worse. In hot weather, our bodies sweat more. Sweating can clog pores and lead to skin irritation. Meanwhile, in the dry and cold temperatures when the air is dry, your skin doesn't shed dead skin cells as efficiently as it should. This can cause your pores to become blocked, leading to breakouts. Acne is not caused by dirt, despite what you may have heard. Washing your face more than twice a day can actually make your acne worse. Acne is not caused by poor hygiene.

Skin tends to become oily and clammy during extremely warm and humid weather. Because of the air's humidity, sweat evaporates more slowly, and the heat makes sebaceous glands work harder. Pimples form as a result of this concoction of conditions.

Sun Exposure

Sun exposure played a noteworthy part in the rate of acne. Some studies showed, people who had more sun exposure as teenagers were less likely to have adult acne. However, sunlight can make acne worse. This is because sunlight dries out your skin and increases oil production. It can also lead to inflammation, which also makes the acne severe. If you have acne-prone skin, you should avoid direct sunlight and use sunscreen when you go outside.

Too Much Sugar

Glycation is a natural chemical reaction that occurs when blood sugar levels rise above what our insulin can handle. Excess sugar in the body can cause this. Collagen and elastin, the components of our skin that keep it "springy," are impacted by glycation. When these two proteins link with sugars, they become weaker, and when these essential building blocks of the skin are damaged, the signs of aging get worse; Wrinkles, sagging, and a dull complexion are all signs of drier and less elastic skin.

Your body quickly converts "simple carbohydrates," such as white flour and refined sugar, into glucose, which then enters the bloodstream. To counteract the spike in glucose, your body responds by producing insulin. This causes inflammation-causing enzymes to attach to your body's collagen.

The causes of acne are many and varied, but the good news is that there are treatments available to help control and manage the condition. If you think your acne may be related to a medication you are taking, or to a hormonal imbalance, talk to your doctor about options for treatment.

In addition, be sure to protect your skin from the sun, and to wash your face no more than twice a day to avoid making your acne worse. But, there are so many external risk factors of acne which can be a reason to cause severe acne levels which will be discussed in the next chapter.

CHAPTER 4

RISK FACTORS AND THINGS TO AVOID

Acne develops for so many reasons, this is what we have already learned. But an overall lifestyle really matters in skin problems. In our daily routine, diet plays the most vital role. It is just like what kind of fuel you use in your vehicle. That will determine the performance of your ride. Similarly, what a person eats has a very massive impact on the happenings of the body.

People with eating habits of spices and oil in their food are most likely to have acne. Spices and oil make some fluids in our skin which can create blockage in the pores. Moreover, people with chubby bodies have a tendency to get oily skin, which ultimately causes blockage in the hair holes of the skin. Then people with a disturbed sleeping cycle are more exposed to hormonal imbalance in their bodies. And acne is most commonly developed due to hormonal changes. As a skincare professional you must advise everyone to decrease their dependency on medications.

People who are less exposed to sunlight have more tendencies to get acne. Sunlight not only prevents acne but also provides vitamin D to our body. So lifestyle matters a lot when it comes to having or avoiding acne.

Bad skin care is also one of the biggest risk factors just like what you put in your body has an impact on your internal health and weight, and what you put on your skin has an impact on your skin's health. You don't need to use a lot of products to have good skin, but you do need to ensure that the products that you're using are well formulated and right for your skin type. In most cases, acne can clear up completely just by consistently having a good skincare routine.

> *According to a 2021 review by Trusted Source, certain foods or diets may have an effect on acne. Consuming certain milk products, like milk and ice cream, seems to worsen acne for some people. Start by eliminating all milk products from your diet for a few weeks to see if your acne improves. On the other hand, consuming too many sugary or processed foods may turn out harmful.*

An unhealthy sleep cycle and sleep deprivation can result in acne as well. As we know, during our sleeping time our body performs all the necessary functions for cell growth, repair, and recovery. So when we don't give enough time to our body for these mandatory functions it results in several skin problems like acne.

Chloracne which is also known as occupational acne is a special type of acne caused by exposure to certain chemicals, such as dioxins. Dioxins are found in pesticides, herbicides, and some industrial chemicals, such as those used in paper mills and wood treatment facilities.

Smoking is really injurious to health, not only for the lungs but also for the skin. It cuts off the oxygen supply to the skin which ultimately results in so many problems and acne is one of them. Along with your wrinkles and rapidly aging skin, smokers often have a sallow, sickly complexion. You begin to take on a pale, splotchy appearance rather than the healthy glow that we all desire as a result of your skin's continuous lack of oxygen and nicotine's restriction of blood vessels, which reduces nutrient and blood flow.

The fact that smoking increases your risk of developing squamous cell skin carcinoma and cataracts in your eyes is another frightening aspect of how smoking affects the skin.

Obesity and being overweight are also risk factors for acne. Studies have shown that people with higher body weight or BMI are at greater risk to get acne. This is because obesity can lead to insulin resistance, which in turn can increase the levels of certain hormones in the body, such as testosterone. And as discussed earlier, an increase in testosterone levels can trigger the development of acne. Chronic inflammatory skin diseases like psoriasis, atopic dermatitis, and skin cancers are caused by obesity and metabolic syndrome, which play a role in their epidemiological prevalence.

Things To Avoid

There are several things that can make your acne problem worse. So it is always better to avoid such things:

- ➢ You should never pop or squeeze your pimples as it will only increase inflammation and make scarring likelier and can be painful too.

- ➢ Avoid touching your face too often as it can transfer the dirt and oil from your hands to your face which can further block your pores and lead to breakouts.

➢ Wearing tight-fitting clothes or headgear can irritate your skin and also trap the sweat and oil on your skin which can clog your pores and lead to breakouts. So, it is always better to wear loose and comfortable clothing.

➢ If you have oily skin, avoid using oil-based makeup products as they can further increase the oiliness of your skin and lead to breakouts. Instead, use water-based or mineral-based makeup products.

➢ Hold the telephone away from the face when talking, as it is likely to contain sebum and skin residue.

➢ Remove makeup with the proper recommended products and cleaners before sleeping. Use epilators, an electric shaver, or sharp safety razors when shaving. Soften the skin and beard with warm soapy water before applying shaving cream.

➢ Keep hair clean, as it collects sebum and skin residue. Avoid oily and greasy hair products, such as those containing cocoa butter.

➢ Avoid anxiety and stress, as it can increase the production of cortisol and adrenaline, which exacerbate acne. Try to keep cool and dry in hot and humid climates, to prevent sweating.

➢ Do not rub your face harshly with a towel after washing it as it can irritate your skin. Instead, pat it dry gently with a soft towel.

➢ If you are using any new skincare product, stop using it immediately if you experience any irritation or redness on your skin, as it may not be suitable for your skin type.

➢ Clean your face no more than twice every day with warm water and mild soap. Few soaps are made especially for acne.

> ➤ Wash hands frequently, especially before applying lotions, creams, or makeup.

> ➤ If you have spectacles, clean them regularly.

Overall, there are a few key things to remember when it comes to acne: avoid dairy and sugary foods, get enough sleep, don't touch your face too much, and use non-comedogenic products. If you do these things, you'll be well on your way to clear skin!

CHAPTER 5
INGREDIENTS THAT CAN HELP

f you want to have complete knowledge about which ingredient you should go with, you need to know the four main stages of acne first. Because treatment and remedies depend upon the severity levels of acne. This chapter will enlighten us about the four levels of acne and the ingredients we should use to stimulate its effect.

In the light of dermatologists and other skin professionals, acne levels can be divided into four levels. These four grade of acne are as follow:

- ➢ Grade 1 - Mild Acne.
- ➢ Grade 2 - Moderate Acne.
- ➢ Grade 3 - Severe Acne.
- ➢ Pustules - Cystic Acne.

Now, let us discuss each one of these levels in detail along with the ingredients which can help.

Grade 1 - Mild Acne

If you are experiencing mild acne it does not mean that you should ignore it because of being a very minor and occasional acne form. No matter what sort of acne you have got, your dissatisfaction with your skin conditions is totally substantial. You ought not to experience serious pimples for your condition to be classified as acne.

Symptoms of mild acne include having periodic minor breakouts, papules, blackheads and whiteheads - all of these appear in mild acne. It is ordinally isolated to fair one or two parts of the face, such as the jawline and chin. It is characterized by 10 or fewer active lesions.

Mild acne can be easily self-diagnosed and it is then easy to use the correct ingredient after knowing the severity level of your acne. You can use over-the-counter (OTC) medicated creams, cleansers, and spot treatments to help address pimples as they pop up. Common ingredients you'll find in acne creams and gels include:

Benzoyl Peroxide

This ingredient is very effective in treating acne because it helps to kill the bacteria which are trapped inside the pores. It also acts as a peeling agent and clears out the dead skin cells which may have accumulated on your face over time. Dead skin cells can act as a breeding ground for bacteria, so by clearing them away you can help to keep your skin clear and blemish-free.

It also helps dry out existing pimples and prevents new ones from forming. Benzoyl peroxide eliminates fatty acids and oils in the skin which works like magic for those who are experiencing acne on oily skin.

Benzoyl peroxide is available in different concentrations, so it's important to start with a lower concentration and increase it gradually as your skin gets used to the ingredient. You can find products containing benzoyl peroxide in the skin care aisle of your local drugstore or beauty store.

Things To Know About Benzoyl Peroxide

While everything has some good as well as bad effects so it is important to have complete know-how about the ingredient before using it. Things that you should already be aware of about this ingredient are:

➤ Expect a bit of dryness and peeling, especially when you first start using it. Because in the initial weeks of its use it can be unexpectedly very disturbing and dry. There is nothing to worry about because it will go away as soon as your skin gets used to it. Those individuals who conquer this time of initial discomfort get the fastest and best results.

➤ You may also experience redness, itchiness, or a burning sensation. This side effect can take a few weeks to go away as your skin needs time to tackle anything.

➤ It can bleach hair, clothing, and bedding, so be careful when applying it to your skin. Try wearing a shirt while applying it. Additionally, it is recommended to use a white washcloth while removing the product from your skin.

➤ Some people find that benzoyl peroxide makes their acne worse before it gets better. If this happens to you, try using a lower concentration or applying it less often.

➤ Benzoyl peroxide can make your skin more sensitive to sunlight, so be sure to use sunscreen when you go outside.

➢ Avoid using it under your eyes, neck, and smile lines because these areas have the most sensitive and delicate tissues which can get irritated and over dry.

➢ The correct way of applying it is to apply it over the complete acne-prone skin. Cover the whole affected area and use it daily. This would help in a way you can not even imagine.

Resorcinol

This ingredient is commonly found in acne treatments which are in the form of lotions and gels. Resorcinol helps to break down blackheads and whiteheads so that they can be removed more easily. It also has antibacterial properties. Resorcinol works by breaking down unpleasant, textured, and solidified skin. It also disinfects the skin to assist fight infection.

It is used in mild form acne and it is recommended to use it topically rather than any other way. Resorcinol topical is utilized to treat torment and itching. It has been used to treat acne, eczema, psoriasis, and many other skin problems for so long.

Best Way To Use

Resorcinol topical does not mean taking it orally but it means to apply directly to your acne-prone skin. Be careful before using it if you are allergic to it or not. Do not apply it on open wounds or on irritated skin.

To know the exact needed dosage for your skin according to its severity level, seek knowledge from its label. Just simply apply it to your acne area and rub it gently until your skin absorbs it completely. Wash your hands after using this ingredient unless you are applying it on your hand too. Store it at room temperature, do not freeze it.

Salicylic Acid

It is an acne-fighting ingredient that is commonly found in cleansers, toners, face creams, and spot treatments. Salicylic acid helps to unclog pores and prevent new pimples from forming. It is a beta-hydroxy acid that has both anti-inflammatory and anti-bacterial properties.

Salicylic acid works by breaking down the bonds between dead skin cells so that they can be removed more easily. It can take a few weeks of use for you to see its full impact. This ingredient also helps exfoliate your skin to prevent pores from getting clogged with acne-causing bacteria.

Things To Know

Every ingredient is recommended according to the current condition of your skin. It is widely used to treat acne, acne spots, acne scars, and melasma (pigmentation). If you have oily skin, it is the best ingredient for you to use.

Before applying it to your skin, wet your acne-prone skin and massage it gently in a circular motion. You may feel a tingling sensation which is normal. Rinse it off with lukewarm water and dry your skin with a clean towel. You can use it 1-2 times daily.

Start with using it once a day and increase the frequency if you see no irritation. If you experience any irritation, redness, or burning sensation, stop using it immediately.

Be more careful if you are going to use this on children because it can cause dryness which can be hard to handle for such sensitive skin like children. It can also interact with certain medications and can cause harmful effects so it is better to have a look at your medications before starting adding this to your daily use.

Sulfur

Sulfur is also known as brimstone. It is a bright yellow element that is found naturally in the earth's crust. It has been used for centuries to treat various skin conditions including acne. Sulfur works by absorbing excess oil, removing dryness, and moisturizing the skin.

Unlike the other ingredients, sulfur does not harm the skin even if it gets used in excess amounts. Sulfur is one of the safest ingredients for all skin types. For those who have sensitive and oily skin, the sulfur ingredient is your savior.

Sulfur has antifungal and keratolytic properties that help to treat acne. Keratolytic substances help in skin shedding, and they may be a successful treatment for dry skin conditions. Sulfur is not liked by everyone because of its pungent smell, but many acne-treating products that contain sulfur do not smell bad. Still, it is always better to smell the product before buying it.

Sulfur gives the best results when used in combination with other acne-treating ingredients. Treating your acne with sulfur as a primary solution will not work the way you expect it to. The biggest advantage of choosing sulfur for your acne treatment is that it is available in a wide range of products. It is not limited to lotions, creams, and ointments only but also it is available in soaps, face wash, and masks. You can also find it in some over-the-counter acne medications.

How To Use Sulfur For Acne?

You can use sulfur in many ways depending on your skin type and sensitivity. As discussed earlier, using sulfur for any type of skin is safe. You can start by using a sulfur soap or cream that has a 2% concentration of sulfur in it.

> ➤ ***Sulfur Foaming Soap*** - If you are using a sulfur soap, wet your face and massage the soap onto your skin for about 30 seconds before rinsing it off. The best-recommended amount is to use it only once a day. Once you wash your face with the sulfur foaming soap in the morning, your morning will begin with less oil, and once you wash your face sometime recently while sleeping, your pores will be clear at night. Moreover, you can have a lot of oil on your skin, do not surpass washing your face more than two times with soap. This will possibly cause more acne.

> ➤ ***Sulfur Cream*** - If you are using a sulfur cream, apply a pea-sized amount of cream on your acne-prone skin and massage it gently towards your skin. Leave it on for about 10 minutes before taking it off. There is no time set to use this cream, you can use it at any time from the 24 hours of the day. If you have oily skin, and you want instant and best results you can increase the concentration of sulfur up to 10%. Many over-the-counter products have 10% sulfur. These products are quite effective in treating acne.

> ➤ ***Sulfur Clay Mask*** - You can make your own sulfur mask at home if you do not want to take any risks for your skin. To make the mask, you will need 1 teaspoon of powdered sulfur, 1 teaspoon of honey, and 1 teaspoon of plain yogurt. Mix all the ingredients together and apply them to your face. Leave it on for about 15 minutes and then take it off.

Meanwhile, some processed clay masks are also available. Masks are always a good go option because it stays for longer in your skin which helps to remove more oil. When you combine sulfur with clay, it gets more powerful because of the clay's dry skin. Utilize this item once a week only. Test out the clay mask from sulfur on your lower arm before you employ it on your sensitive skin. In case, you have got any skin sort, you can either apply the mask to your whole face or on the other oily areas.

Splash your face first, then dry your face with a clean towel. Avoid applying the mask to your eyebrows, lips, and eyes. Let it stay on your time for the time which is mentioned on the masking label, it's always better to follow the instructions provided on the label.

Azelaic Acid

Azelaic acid is an organic compound that can be derived from whole-grain cereals. This acid is also found in animal products. Azelaic acid is an antiseptic ingredient that is so extreme against acne bacteria that it's an OTC choice for treating cystic acne and has been considered to be nearly as successful as Accutane.

Azelaic acid works by inhibiting the growth of keratinocytes, which are the cells that make up the outer layer of your skin. It has a combination of all the anti-bacterial, anti-fungal, and anti-inflammatory properties. These properties make it an ideal ingredient for acne treatment. Indeed even though azelaic acid could be an effective fix, it is gentle on the skin and secures all skin sorts.

Acne Scars - Azelaic acid is not only helpful for acne but also for acne scars. Azelaic acid can help in the fading of post-inflammatory hyperpigmentation (PIH). PIH is a type of scar that is caused by the overproduction of melanin. Melanin is a pigment that gives your skin its color. When there is an overproduction of melanin, it can lead to the darkening of the skin.

Azelaic acid works by inhibiting the production of melanin. It does this by inhibiting the activity of tyrosinase, which is an enzyme that is responsible for the production of melanin. Azelaic acid is also an antioxidant, and it can help to repair the damage that has been caused by free radicals.

Removes Dead Skin Cells - Azelaic acid also assists in removing dead skin cells from the surface of the skin. It does this by increasing the turnover of skin cells. When there is an increase in the turnover of skin cells, the dead skin cells are shed from the surface of the skin at a faster rate. The scientific reason behind this process is that like other ingredients it also has keratolytic properties.

Hyperpigmentation - Azelaic acid can also be used to treat hyperpigmentation. Hyperpigmentation is the darkening of the skin. A pilot study from 2011 showed azelaic acid can treat skin break out whereas evening out hyperpigmentation is activated by acne. Advance research on the skin of color has moreover shown that azelaic acid is safe and sound and useful for this use.

Rosacea - Azelaic acid is often used to treat rosacea. Rosacea is a chronic skin condition that causes redness and inflammation on the face. Azelaic acid helps by reducing redness and inflammation by inhibiting the growth of keratinocytes.

Clinical studies illustrate that azelaic acid gel can ceaselessly progress the appearance of swelling and obvious blood vessels caused by rosacea.

Prevents Future Acne Breakouts - Azelaic acid could be a comedolytic, meaning it anticipates future whiteheads and blackheads from forming. By keeping pores clean, whiteheads and blackheads would not create from an overabundance of oil or dead skin cell build-up. FYI, salicylic acid and benzoyl peroxide are also comedolytics.

Side Effects

Azelaic acid is generally well tolerated. But it can cause some side effects including:

- ➢ Skin dryness or redness.
- ➢ Peeling of skin at the location of the application.
- ➢ Fever.
- ➢ Burning or shivering on your skin.
- ➢ Hives and itching.

Grade 2 - Moderate Acne

In moderate acne, you will have a lot of papules and pustules as well as a few nodules. Your acne will cover a large area of your face, back, or chest. You may also start to experience scarring at this stage. There will be more blemishes.

In this grade of acne papules when squeezed, no fluid will come out. Pustules when pressed, yellow color pus will come out some of the time blended with blood.   If you continue to experience symptoms after using OTC acne treatments for several weeks, you may want to consider reaching out for professional treatment. A dermatologist or other healthcare professional can prescribe medications that may help reduce your symptoms and prevent scarring. If you have moderate acne, a dermatologist may recommend:

Antibiotics

Antibiotics means either a pill you take by mouth or a gel or lotion you apply to your skin. Their job is to kill the bacteria that contribute to acne. Two of the most common and major antibiotics used to treat acne are:

- ➢ Erythromycin
- ➢ Clindamycin

Erythromycin

Erythromycin is an antibiotic medicine used for acne cures. Its active ingredient is erythromycin whereas excipients are propylene glycol and ethanol 96%. Patients with known hypersensitivity to erythromycin and other macrolide anti-microbials or propylene glycol should avoid using this medicine.

Erythromycin is a macrolide antibiotic. It interferes with bacterial protein union by authoritative to 50S subunit or ribosomes of touchy organisms.

- It reduces the follicular porphyrin fluorescence and free fatty acids levels of skin lipids.

- It also inhibits the bacteria from producing the protein which is essential for the bacteria. In the absence of those proteins, bacteria can not grow and acne will not get initiated.

- It does not specifically slaughter the bacteria but takes off them incapable to extend in numbers. The remaining microscopic organisms inevitably die or are devastated by the immune system.

- By controlling the bacterial growth, the inflammatory system gets in control and the skin gets time to heal.

The liquid erythromycin is for external use only. You can not inject it or take it orally. Do not make it in contact with your eyes, mouth, and the inside of your nose. Do not use it if you are allergic to any of the ingredients present in it. Do not use any other oral medication for acne while you are using this.

Clindamycin

It is used to treat infections with anaerobic bacteria and certain types of microorganisms. These bacteria are the ones that don't need oxygen to grow and multiply. In general, clindamycin is a member of the lincomycin antibiotic family. Clindamycin phosphate is its active ingredient whereas cetyl alcohol and propylene glycol are excipients.

Clindamycin is a topical antibiotic that is successful at diminishing the side effects and appearance of acne. Clindamycin has both bacteriostatic and bactericidal properties, meaning that it works to halt microbes from increasing and murdering destructive cells straightforwardly. It can also be used before dental procedures to prevent infections in people with heart conditions who can not use antibiotics.

Oral Contraceptives

Oral contraceptives are birth control pills that can also help reduce the size and number of pimples in women. The ingredients in the birth control pills can change, so you should make it beyond any doubt your medicines contain the proper blend of hormones. The hormones in these pills can slow down the amount of oil produced by your skin.

The pills diminish the circulation of androgens, which diminishes the circulation of sebum. These contraceptives must contain both estrogen and progestin to be successful against acne. The mini pill, which contains only progestin, can really prompt an expansion in pimple breakouts.

Progestin-just pills are not a decent alternative for ladies who smoke. The danger of stroke and coronary illness is too high for ladies who smoke and utilize just progestin pills as a type of contraception. If you have side effects from one brand of pill, you may have the capacity to switch to another brand. A few ladies find that their skin clears up when they change pills.

You'll need to take oral contraceptives for a few months before you start to see an improvement in your skin. It might take up to a year for your skin to clear completely.

A 2012 review looked at 31 trials involving the use of birth control as an acne treatment. After looking at six new trials, the authors concluded that all combination birth control pills treated noninflammatory and inflammatory acne.

Some of the pills which are approved by the Food and Drug Administration (FDA) for the treatment of acne are:

➢ Beyaz.

➢ Estrostep Fe.

➢ Ortho Tri-cyclen.

➢ Yaz.

The most common side effect of oral contraceptives is nausea. All of the common and serious side effects include:

➢ Headaches.

➢ Weight gain.

➢ Mood swings.

➢ Breast tenderness.

➢ Spotting between periods.

➢ Blood clots.

➢ Heart attack.

➢ Stroke.

➢ Liver tumors.

Some women stop taking oral contraceptives because of the side effects. But the side effects usually go away after a few months. If they don't, talk to your doctor about switching to another brand of pill.

Grade 3 - Severe Acne

Severe acne is when you have 50 to 100 pimples. You might also have larger pimples called nodules and cysts. These can be painful and leave scars. Severe acne can happen at any age, but it's most common in teenagers and young adults. Since the lesions happen close to each other, they can spread and consolidate with each other and appear like a crop.

Severe acne is hard to cure as compared to other grades. You might have to try more than one type of treatment before you find what works for you. Often, a combination of treatments is the most successful approach. Topical treatment is not enough at this grade. Professional help and visits to dermatologists become necessary.

Corticosteroid Injections

Corticosteroid injections are a type of anti-inflammatory medication. They can help reduce the size of large pimples quickly. Injections are usually reserved for people with nodular or cystic acne — severe forms of acne that cause large, painful bumps.

According to the Journal of the American Academy of Dermatology, cortisone shots' zit-zapping sorcery is real. Corticosteroid shots are an effective treatment for individual, large acne nodules when injected directly into the pimple, and they can rapidly reduce pain and flatten the pimple.

Everything You Need to Know

A cortisone shot is a "quick fix" for acne because it immediately reduces inflammation. Corticosteroid injections are usually safe when administered by a board-certified dermatologist or other qualified healthcare professional.

It is an injection of a synthetic hormone. These injections can be used on any part of the body including the face. The doctors usually used to inject the injection directly into the inflamed cysts or nodules which instantly get better within a few days.

Corticosteroid injections are relatively inexpensive, especially when compared to the cost of some oral acne medications. Dermatologists can offer a viable alternative for people with severe nodular or cystic acne who cannot tolerate or have not responded to other forms of treatment, such as oral antibiotics or isotretinoin.

Risks and Side Effects of Corticosteroid Injections

There is always the risk of infection whenever the skin is broken. To help reduce the risk, the injection site is first cleansed with an antiseptic solution.

Corticosteroid injections may cause temporary depressions in the skin (called "dells") or lighten the skin around the injection site. Injecting corticosteroids too frequently can also lead to thinning of the skin. You should wait for at least 6 weeks before having an injection on the same spot.

As with any type of medication, there is always the potential for side effects. The most common side effects of corticosteroid injections include:

1. Temporary pain at the injection site.
2. Redness.

3. Swelling.

4. Lightening or darkening of the skin around the injection site.

5. Temporary bumps (called "wheals").

6. Skin infection.

7. Tearing of the skin.

8. Allergic reactions.

9. Worsening of acne if used persistently.

Oral Isotretinoin (Accutane)

Isotretinoin is an oral medication used to treat severe nodular or cystic acne. It is usually restricted to people who have not responded to other forms of treatment, such as antibiotics or corticosteroid injections.

Isotretinoin has five biologically important metabolites. Four of these are known to be active: 4-oxo-isotretinoin, retinoic acid (tretinoin), cis-acneclidine, and trans-acneclidine. The fifth metabolite has not been identified.

Brand names for isotretinoin include Absorica®, Amnesteem®, Claravis®, Myorisan®, and Zenatane™. Some people refer to this medication as Accutane®. This is a brand of isotretinoin that is no longer available.

Benefits Of Isotretinoin

Isotretinoin can be very effective in treating acne. If no other treatment or medication is working for you, isotretinoin can be an option.

This medication can dramatically improve the appearance and texture of your skin. It can also reduce the size of your pores, which can make your skin shine and creates a glow on your skin overall.

Isotretinoin can also help prevent future breakouts. Studies have shown that people who take isotretinoin have a lower risk of developing new acne. It moreover results in a noteworthy lessening of sebum production.

Side Effects Of Isotretinoin

Like every other medication, isotretinoin also has some side effects.

- ➤ **Dryness:** You may experience dryness of the skin, lips, and eyes while taking isotretinoin. You can use a lip balm or moisturizer to help with the dryness. Drink plenty of water and avoid sunlight to prevent dehydration.

- ➤ **Joint and muscle pain:** Joint and muscle pain is most likely to occur when you start taking isotretinoin. Be sure to take breaks throughout the day and do some light stretching exercises to help reduce the pain.

- ➤ **Birth defects:** Do not take isotretinoin if you are pregnant or may become pregnant during treatment. If you get pregnant while taking isotretinoin, stop taking it right away and call your doctor.

- ➤ **Depression and suicide:** Some people taking isotretinoin have had thoughts about hurting themselves or putting an end to their own lives (suicide). Some people have ended their lives while taking isotretinoin. So be very careful with the dosage of medicine and be calm with your treatment process.

- ➤ **Other major diseases can occur:** People with IBD have an increased risk of developing IBD while taking isotretinoin. Likewise, the risk of having pancreatitis and liver diseases also increases.

Grade 4 - Cystic Acne

Cystic acne is the most severe form of acne. It occurs when oil and dead skin cells build up in the pores and form deep, painful bumps called cysts. Cysts are large, red, and inflamed. They can be very tender to touch. In this grade of acne, there are blisters that look like a bubble or a huge rankle. The measure of a cyst can be around half a centimeter in distance across. This cyst contains pus inside. But the nodules do not contain pus inside them.

Cystic acne is more common in teenage boys than girls. But it can occur in people of any age. It often runs in families. People with cystic acne may also have regular acne. Treatment usually lasts for 4 to 6 months.

There are a lot of over-the-counter and prescription medications available for the treatment of cystic acne. But not every medication is suitable for everyone. Your overall health and skin damage level determine which treatment will work best for you.

Doxycycline

Doxycycline is a very popular oral antibiotic to treat cystic acne. Everyone has bacteria on their skin; it is normal. In fact, your skin is home to around 1,000 different kinds of bacteria.

Doxycycline treats acne by destroying the skin's bacteria, preventing them from causing inflammation. Doxycycline also helps acne by reducing skin inflammation.

It has a good safety record, is highly effective, and has been used in dermatology for decades. In addition, doxycycline reduces inflammation by inhibiting the activity of inflammatory blood cells and enzymes and messengers that contribute to acne-related skin inflammation and irritation.

Even though you may have been persuaded to purchase this medication to treat your persistent acne, we must inform you that doxycycline is not available over the counter. It's actually a prescription drug that comes in tablet or capsule form for oral consumption. Therefore, you must first get a prescription from your dermatologist before you can use this.

Side Effects Caused By Doxycycline

As with all medications, there are potential side effects associated with doxycycline. The most common ones include:

Heartburn also known as acidity: Is caused when the stomach's acid comes up through the esophagus and causes a burning sensation in the chest.

In some severe cases, it can cause esophageal inflammation and esophageal or gastric ulcers.

General Things To Keep In Mind While Using Doxycycline

- Doxycycline should be taken with a full glass of water.
- It is advisable to take doxycycline with food or milk to avoid an upset stomach.
- You should not lie down for at least 10 minutes after taking this medication.
- If you miss a dose, take it as soon as possible. If it is almost time for your next dose, skip the missed dose and go back to your regular dosing schedule. Do not take 2 doses at once.
- Store this medication at room temperature away from light and moisture. Do not store it in the bathroom. Keep all medications away from children and pets.

CHAPTER 6

NATURAL INGREDIENTS FOR TREATING ACNE

There are many home remedies for acne that have been passed down from generation to generation. Some of these remedies are effective, while others are not. The effectiveness of a home remedy for acne depends on the individual and the severity of their acne.

Many people believe that home remedies are a better option than conventional treatments because they are natural and have fewer side effects. However, there is no scientific evidence to support this claim.

The majority of people either choose to live with acne or, out of frustration, turn to chemical or medication treatments that frequently have negative side effects or do not work at all. Home remedies work for all the same reasons that medical treatments work: they kill bacteria, dry up oil, and reduce inflammation. There is no restriction to using it in any grade of acne you can use it at any level.

Most home remedies for acne call for common kitchen ingredients that can be found in any grocery store.

Apple Cider Vinegar

Apple cider vinegar (ACV) is a common home remedy for treating heartburn, controlling one's appetite, and getting rid of moles. Test-tube studies show that vinegar can kill some kinds of bacteria. This is because it contains a lot of acetic acids, which gives it its acidity. Additionally, apple cider vinegar contains a number of other organic acids, which are lactic acid, gallic acid, chlorogenic acid, and protocatechuic acid.

Acne scarring can also be helped by using lactic acid, but the small amount of diluted ACV is unlikely to have a significant impact. It also provides some benefits such as: reducing hyperpigmentation, chemically exfoliates, and restoring pH balance to the skin.

Before applying vinegar to your skin, the concentrations of organic acids need to be significantly diluted. So there are different ways by which you can use apple cider vinegar safely.

Make ACV Toner

For making apple cider vinegar toner you need one part of apple cider vinegar, two parts of water, 1 tsp of rose water, 2-3 drops of essential oil (lavender or chamomile recommended), and 1 tsp of witch hazel (if you have oily skin). You can also add a little bit of honey to it for taste.

Apply this mixture to the acne by soaking a cotton ball in apple cider vinegar and applying it to the affected area. Leave it on for 10-15 minutes and then wash it off with water. Do this twice daily for the best results.

Make a DIY Facial Cleanser

ACV can also be used to make a facial cleanser. For this, you need 1 part of ACV, 2 parts of water, and 1 tsp of aloe vera gel (optional). Mix all these ingredients together and store them in a clean bottle. To use it, take some cleanser on your palm and massage it all over your face for a minute. Wash it off with lukewarm water and pat dry. Use this cleanser once or twice daily as per your convenience.

Use It As An Exfoliant

ACV is great at gently exfoliating skin because it contains malic acid. Take a bath with a cup of apple cider vinegar and warm water for the best results. To achieve soft skin, all you need is 15 minutes.

Use It As A Spot Treatment

Dab some apple cider vinegar onto a cotton ball and apply it only to the pimple. Leave it on overnight and rinse it off in the morning. You should see a reduction in swelling and redness. If you have sensitive skin, avoid using ACV directly on your skin as it can cause burning and irritation.

Tea-Tree Oil

Tea-tree oil is made up of the leaves of the Australian tree with the same name used to make tea tree oil. It has been used as traditional medicine by Aboriginal Australians for many centuries. Medications containing 5% benzoyl peroxide may not be as effective as tea tree oil gels containing 5% tea tree oil.

Tea tree oil was applied twice daily to the participants' faces for 12 weeks in a 2017 study, according to Trusted Source. The researchers came to the conclusion that, without serious side effects, tea tree oil can "significantly improve" mild to moderate acne. However, this study had only 14 participants and did not meet other quality standards for research.

It is a common and inexpensive essential oil that is frequently used in treatments for hair and skin. This oil is a well-known anti-bacterial treatment for acne that also works well on the skin. It is qualified to treat a variety of conditions, including acne, cold sores, hair loss, and skin blisters.

When applied topically, tea tree oil can speed up acne healing. It has been demonstrated to be effective, but due to its potency, it should only be used sparingly. Additionally, it may not be able to be tolerated by those with sensitive skin. Tea tree oil should be stopped immediately if it causes any side effects.

<u>How To Use Tea-tree Oil For Acne</u>

1. 12 drops of carrier oil are combined with one to two drops of tea tree oil. However, use any additional oils with caution on your face. Acne can be made worse by using any oily product.

2. Do a small patch test on the inside of your elbow with diluted tea tree oil before applying it to your face. Itching, redness, swelling, and burning are symptoms of skin sensitivity or an allergic reaction.

3. Wash your face with an acne-prone skin-friendly gentle cleanser and pat it dry before applying the oil.

4. Apply diluted tea tree oil to your skin by dabbing it on with a cotton round or pad.

5. Let it dry. Use your usual moisturizer as a follow-up.

6. Morning and evening, repeat.

Green Tea

Catechins are plant-based compounds found in green tea. Epigallocatechin gallate (EGCG) is one of the catechin compounds found in green tea. Acne could be prevented or treated with EGCG's significant anti-inflammatory, antibiotic, and antioxidant properties. It is rich in antioxidants, which can fight free radicals and prevent inflammation. These benefits may extend to the skin, making green tea a potential home remedy for acne.

A small 2013 study found that applying a 2% green tea lotion to the skin improved acne by 25% after six weeks. The lotion was also well tolerated by the participants.

Another 2015 study looked at the effects of green tea extract on acne. The researchers found that the extract had a significant effect in reducing the number of pimples in people with mild to moderate acne.

How to Use Green Tea

There are a few different options available to you if you are willing to give green tea a shot for acne. A method based on trial and error might be the most effective. Keep in mind that green tea for the skin does not have a specific dosing recommendation.

Green tea facial spritz - In a spray bottle with a top, combine three parts of water with one part of green tea. After cleansing your face and applying moisturizer, spritz the solution on it. Let it get dry for 10 - 15 minutes and then clean your face. Do not do it more than twice a week.

Green tea toner - Two cups of boiling water are combined with one and a half teaspoons of green tea leaves. Before straining the leaves, let the mixture steep for three minutes. Once it has cooled, use a cotton ball to apply the toner to your face. Do this once a day after cleansing your face.

Green tea mask - First, make a green tea paste by combining two tablespoons of water and one teaspoon of green tea leaves. Also, add some Aleo vera and honey. Mix it well until you get the desired quality of the paste. It should be applied to your face and left on for ten minutes. Rinse your face with lukewarm water after that. Two times a week, do this.

As a spot treatment - After boiling two cups of water, turn off the heat. Then, add the leaves of one and a half teaspoons of green tea. Allow it to sit for three minutes before taking the leaves out. Give the solution time to cool and then put it in a clean cotton ball. Apply green tea to your pimples. Leave it on for 10 minutes, and then rinse your face with water.

Drink Green Tea - You can also reap the potential benefits of green tea, including those for the skin, by drinking it every day as part of a healthy lifestyle. Just avoid adding sugar, as this can negate the beneficial effects. Two to three cups of green tea can be consumed in a day either hot or cold.

<u>Few More Tips</u>

➢ Choose organic green teas with fewer processing steps if you have acne-prone skin. This will lower the likelihood of being contaminated with additional harmful chemicals that could aggravate acne.

➢ Before using green tea on your face, perform a patch test on a small area of skin, such as the inside of your elbow, to check for allergic reactions.

> ➢ When using green tea as a home remedy for acne, be patient. Results may not be evident for several weeks or even longer.

Omega-3 Fatty Acids

Omega-3 fatty acids are beneficial not only to the body but also to the skin. Fish like salmon, mackerel, and herring contain these fatty acids. They can also be found in some oils made from plants, like hemp oil and flaxseed oil.

According to the researchers, these fatty acids reduce inflammation by lowering IGF-1 levels and stimulating the body to produce the anti-inflammatory prostaglandins E1 and E3 and leukotriene B5. Acne is known to be caused by IGF-1.

Inflammation in the body is reduced by omega-3 fatty acids. This includes skin inflammation. A placebo or omega-3 supplements were given to acne sufferers in one study. After 12 weeks, the group that took the omega 3 supplements had significantly fewer pimples.

Dietary fatty acids are incorporated into the cell membranes by the body. A cell's membrane can hold water when it is healthy. Cells in the skin become hydrated and supple as a result. Additionally, we are aware that Omega 3 lowers inflammation while Omega 6 raises it. Our bodies function best when the two are in balance, but the average Western diet contains 20 times more Omega 6 than Omega 3.

Your skin cell membranes can't properly replicate if you don't have enough of any of the Omegas, so they can't take in nutrients or get rid of toxins. Every day, as our old cells die and new ones grow, skin cells reproduce themselves. But when you heal something, like acne or a wound, skin cells reproduce at a much faster rate. The membranes of those new cells must be healthy and properly replicated.

How to Use Omega 3 Fatty Acids

There are a few different ways you can use omega-3 fatty acids to help treat your acne.

Omega 3 supplements: Omega 3 supplements can be taken as pills. To avoid side effects like stomach upset, start with a lower dose and gradually increase it over time. The usual daily dose of around 1000 mg is what is recommended. Look for concentrations of at least 60%.

Fish Oil Omega-3 Supplements - You can also get omega-3 fatty acids by eating fish. Salmon, mackerel, and herring are all good sources. Cold-water fish are the best since they contain more beneficial oils. Fish oil supplements usually come in capsules or liquids. The fatty acids in fish oil can help to:

- ➤ Stimulate the production of anti-inflammatory agents.
- ➤ Reduce sebum production.
- ➤ Soothe the skin by reducing inflammation.

Flaxseed Oil Omega-3 Supplements - Flaxseed oil is another good source of omega-3s. Due to a chemical known as lignan, flaxseed oil can also be used to treat acne. This chemical is found in plants and is referred to as phytoestrogen, which means that it behaves similarly to the body's hormone estrogen.

As a result, it is believed that lignan and other phytoestrogens like isoflavonoids and coumestans aid in reproduction, reduce inflammation, and prevent some cancers. In addition to reducing acne-related inflammation, lignan may also lessen the effects of hormonal imbalances that contribute to or cause acne.

Hemp Oil Omega-3 Supplements - The high content of omega-6 and omega-3 fatty acids in hemp seed oil contributes to its skin-benefitting properties. These nutrients can help treat atopic dermatitis and other skin conditions.

After 20 weeks, one randomized, single-blind crossover study demonstrated that dietary hempseed oil reduced clinical atopic dermatitis symptoms and appearance.

Hemp oil has anti-aging properties in addition to being soothing and moisturizing for the skin. Hemp oil can aid in the reduction of wrinkles and fine lines as well as the prevention of aging-related signs. The linoleic and oleic acids in hemp oil can't be made by the body, but they can help keep skin healthy and prevent aging, so it's important to include them in your diet.

Topical Application - Omega-3 fatty acids can also be applied to the skin directly. Fish oil or flaxseed oil-based products can be used to accomplish this. Creams, lotions, and serums are examples of these products. Meanwhile, it is not the most liked way to treat acne, oral capsules are preferred.

Jojoba Oil

Similar to sebum, the oil that our skin naturally produces, jojoba oil is a type of oil. Jojoba oil can help regulate sebum production when applied to the skin. Acne breakouts may be reduced as a result of this. Because it is non-comedogenic, jojoba oil will not clog pores. Additionally, jojoba oil is non-irritating and hypoallergenic, making it an excellent option for people with sensitive skin.

Research upholds that jojoba oil is gainful in regarding skin break out as fixing and all alone. A clay and jojoba oil facial mask was found to be effective in treating mild acne and skin lesions in a 2012 German study. Acne, inflammation, and lesions were significantly reduced in participants who used jojoba oil masks two to three times per week. According to a case study, jojoba oil worked as a herbal remedy to alleviate acne symptoms.

Jojoba oil should only be purchased from reputable businesses. The oil that is labeled "unrefined" indicates that it has not been filtered and does not contain any additives. The oil that has been refined may have been bleached or processed. Additionally, look for jojoba oil with low oleic acid content. On skin that is more sensitive, oleic acid can clog pores and cause breakouts.

Oil can be made from the jojoba plant's nuts. Because it is so mild, jojoba oil can be mixed with other essential oils as a carrier oil. It can also be used by itself. Jojoba oil is a humectant ingredient. This indicates that it assists in maintaining the skin's hydration by attracting water to the top layer. This may aid in the prevention of bacterial infections, acne, and dandruff.

<u>How To Use Jojoba Oil For Acne</u>

As we have already illustrated that jojoba oil can benefit the skin without clogging pores. It is used in a variety of commercial products which can use include:

➢ **As a makeup remover** - Use a makeup sponge or napkin and a small amount of jojoba oil to thoroughly and gently remove your makeup.It's important to remove your makeup before you go to bed because leaving it on while you sleep can cause breakouts. Gently massage a small amount of the oil onto your face with your fingertips to break up makeup and sebum. Rinse thoroughly with warm water.

➤ **As a clay mask** - The skin can be soothed and nourished by applying a jojoba oil mask. Simply add a few drops of jojoba oil to a clay mask you've made or bought from the store. Rinse the mixture off your face with warm water after applying it to your face and letting it sit for 15 minutes. After you wash it off, your skin may appear red, so you might want to avoid doing this during the day.

➤ **As a moisturizer** - In a pump bottle that is empty, thoroughly shake jojoba oil and aloe vera gel in proportions equal to 1. Rub your hands together with two to three squirts in your hand. After that, apply the mixture to your skin with a light press and wait 15 seconds for it to absorb. Remove any excess and reapply as necessary. Jojoba oil is a moisturizer that can last up to 24 hours. After you apply it, your skin will appear more hydrated and plump.

➤ **As an in-shower treatment** - You can use jojoba oil as a natural in-shower body moisturizer. Add a small amount of jojoba oil to your regular body wash. Gently massage the mixture into your skin in circular motions and wash it off during your shower. Your skin will feel soft, smooth, and hydrated after using this method.

Coconut Oil

One of the many wonderful applications of this versatile, naturally occurring oil is the discovery that it can be used to treat acne. Most of the medium-chain fatty acids in coconut oil are MCFAs. Capric, caproic, and caprylic MCFAs are also found in coconut oil.

Although not as potent as lauric acid, some of these are effective against acne-causing bacteria. Acne can be treated with this natural and effective treatment. It has antimicrobial properties that can assist in eliminating acne-causing bacteria. Additionally, coconut oil can reduce redness and soothe inflamed skin.

A study published in the Journal of Dermatology found that coconut oil was effective in treating xerosis, which is a type of skin inflammation. Coconut oil can help combat bacteria while alleviating dry skin.

Unfortunately, people with extremely oily skin may not benefit from coconut oil. Coconut oil is a white solid when it is cool. It turns into a clear liquid when heated. Coconut oil is a very durable oil that doesn't go rancid even after being stored for a long time and exposed to extreme temperatures.

Therefore, when you use coconut oil to treat acne, you not only give your skin the ammunition it needs to fight off acne-causing agents (antimicrobials), but you also protect your skin from additional assaults (antioxidants), hydrate it to aid in healing, and give it a boost of hydration. Additionally, coconut oil contains Vitamin E, a natural antioxidant that protects the skin from environmental toxins and skin cancer. Vitamin E can be kept potent for a long time in coconut oil, which is a great source of vitamin E.

How To Use Coconut Oil For Acne

Coconut oil can be used in two primary ways to treat or prevent acne on the skin: It can be consumed or applied topically (to the skin's surface). Both are options but in any of the options, it is important to check if you are using virgin or organic coconut oil.

Cold-pressed virgin or extra virgin coconut oil is coconut oil that is extracted without the use of chemicals, compounds, or additives. This ensures that the oil maintains its original chemical composition and all of its beneficial properties for health.

Topical Coconut Oil With A Steam Bath

This is an easy and effective way to open your pores and let the coconut oil penetrate deep into your skin. This method can be used 1–2 times per week.

- Start by heating a pot of water on the stove until it reaches a boiling point.
- Carefully pour the hot water into a bowl.
- Add 3–4 drops of lavender or tea tree essential oil to the water.
- Cover your head with a towel and lean over the bowl.
- Allow the steam to open your pores for 5–10 minutes.
- Gently pat your face dry with a clean towel.
- Apply a thin layer of coconut oil to your face and neck and leave the oil on for 20 minutes.
- Clean your face and apply a natural moisturizer to your skin after you are done.

Oral Consumption Of Coconut Oil

Coconut oil can be consumed as a natural acne remedy. Coconut oil's fatty acids have the potential to aid in the elimination of harmful yeast and bacteria that can cause breakouts.

Simply include between one and two tablespoons of organic virgin coconut oil in your daily diet. It can be added to yogurt, oatmeal, and smoothies. It can also be used to prepare meals in place of other cooking oils. Consuming coconut oil for at least three months will help you see the greatest improvement in your acne.

<u>Topical Warmed Coconut Oil</u>

All you need to do is to put a teaspoon of cool, solid coconut oil in your palm and use that as your guide. In between your palms, warm it. After that, you can rub the coconut oil into the skin in circular motions directly onto the problem areas. For additional hydrating and acne-fighting benefits, you can wrap any remaining coconut oil around your face.

Aloe Vera Gel

The succulent family of plants includes aloe vera. It has thick, serrated leaves and grows in the wild. Aloe vera leaves contain a clear, sticky gel that is applied topically to soothe burned or irritated skin. Aloe vera gel has many benefits for the skin. It can be used to heal wounds, moisturize the skin, and treat acne.

Aloe vera gel is made up of 97% water and 3% solid matter. Solid matter consists of various minerals, enzymes, vitamins, sugars, and amino acids. Aloe vera gel also contains salicylic acid, which is a compound that has been shown to have anti-inflammatory and antibacterial properties.

Gibberellins and glycol-proteins are known to be present in aloe vera. These ingredients encourage skin repair and growth. Additionally, aloe vera contains gibberellins and auxin.By encouraging cell growth, these hormones aid in wound healing.

Aloe vera may increase the immune system's response to inflammation, which may reduce the appearance of acne scarring, according to a 2009 article in the International Journal of Natural Therapy.

Aloesin, a compound found in aloe vera, may reduce acne scar hyperpigmentation. Aloesin helps reduce melanin, a darker pigment that can make acne scars look worse. Gels containing aloe vera can be found in most pharmacies and online. Nevertheless, not all of them are made for the face. Look for words like these on labels:

> ➢ Non-comedogenic
> ➢ Fragrance-free
> ➢ Suitable for the face and body

How to Use Aloe Vera Gel for Acne

When combined with standard acne treatments, aloe vera has been shown to have positive effects. Try these at home if you have mild to moderate acne and are looking for a gentle way to soothe your skin.

Topical Pure Aloe Vera Gel

Aloe vera can be used on its own to achieve the desired results. You can increase the blood flow to your skin and eliminate harmful bacteria by purchasing pure aloe vera and applying it generously to your face instead of a cleanser. You can also use aloe to treat specific areas of acne breakouts, apply it, let it sit overnight, and then wash it off the next day to ease redness and irritation.

Aloe and Lemon Juice Face Mask

Ingredients:

> ➢ 1 tablespoon of fresh aloe vera gel.
> ➢ 1 teaspoon of freshly squeezed lemon juice.
> ➢ 2 drops of lavender essential oil (optional).

Instructions:

- ➤ Combine all ingredients in a small bowl and mix until they are fully combined.
- ➤ Apply the mask to your face using clean fingers or a cotton pad, avoiding the eye area.
- ➤ Leave the mask on for 10-15 minutes and then rinse it off with water.
- ➤ Finish by applying your favorite moisturizer.

Lavender oil has antimicrobial properties and can be used to treat acne scars; however, it is not necessary for this recipe. If you decide to use it, make sure to only add a couple of drops as lavender oil can be irritating to the skin if used in too high of a concentration.

Aloe Vera Spray

Because it is less likely to irritate sensitive skin, this is an excellent choice. It can be used as a toner, makeup remover, or even to set your makeup.

Ingredients:

- ➤ 1/4 cup of aloe vera gel.
- ➤ 3/4 cup of rose water (or distilled water).
- ➤ 1/2 teaspoon of glycerin.

Instructions:

- ➤ Mix all of the ingredients in a small bowl or jar until well combined.
- ➤ Fill a spray bottle that is clean and empty with the mixture.
- ➤ Simply spray the spray onto your face whenever you need to refresh your skin or take off your makeup to use it.

Because aloe vera can dry out the skin, you should moisturize your skin after using any of these treatments. Look for a moisturizer that doesn't contain oil if you have oily skin; If you have dry skin, choose one with glycerin or hyaluronic acid in it.

Honey

Honey is a natural humectant, which means it helps retain moisture in the skin. Enzyme activity, plant matter, and live bacteria combine to produce honey in its natural state, a potent ingredient with hundreds of useful applications. Honey controls the production of candida Albicans, a fungus that can cause acne.

The effectiveness of manuka honey as an acne treatment has been studied and found to be significantly higher than that of other well-known products. For the honey to be effective, it must still contain its beneficial bacteria. Your immune system will be activated, and blemishes and inflammation will be alleviated.

However, because honey is an exfoliant, applying it to your face can get rid of dull-looking dead skin cells. This may show skin that is brighter. Honey can be applied as a paste at the site of your scars everyday or every other day as a spot treatment for scars.

The glucose oxidase immediately transforms into hydrogen peroxide when honey is applied to the skin. Benzoyl peroxide, which is found in products to treat acne as discussed earlier, performs the same function as hydrogen peroxide.

Honey is best for acne that is red and inflamed.It aids in the removal of acne impurities. Other compounds in honey, such as fatty acids, vitamin B, peptides, amino acids, antioxidants, and others, have a calming effect on acne. These calming substances reduce acne's redness and fade scars after treatment.

How To Use Honey For Acne

Like other ingredients, acne works best when honey is mixed with other items. Some of the ingredients you can mix and use are:

Honey And Yogurt Mask

Ingredients:

- ➢ 1 tablespoon of Manuka honey.
- ➢ 2 tablespoons of plain yogurt.

Instructions:

- ➢ Mix all the ingredients collectively until they are combined and smooth.
- ➢ Apply the mask that you just made to your face, and be careful with the eye and lips.
- ➢ Leave it on for 10-15 minutes and then rinse it off.

This mask is as simple to practice as it sounds, but it provides plenty of benefits. You do not need to rush to pharmacies and buy expensive products for your skincare. Just go in the kitchen and get the glow!

Raw Honey, Lemon Juice, And Baking Soda

Ingredients:

- ➢ 1 tablespoon of raw honey.
- ➢ 1 teaspoon of freshly squeezed lemon juice.
- ➢ 1/4 teaspoon of baking soda.

Instructions:

> Keep mixing these ingredients together until it appears like a fine paste.

> Splash your face with water first and then gently apply the mixture to your skin with your fingertips very gently.

> Let it set for 5-10 minutes and then wash the pack once it is dry.

Repeat this process 2-3 times a week for the best results. While this may sound like a weird combination, these three ingredients work together to brighten your skin, reduce scars, and fight acne. The citric acid in lemon juice acts as an astringent to help dry out pimples. Raw honey is a natural antibiotic that helps heal the skin and reduces redness. Baking soda is an exfoliant that helps remove dead skin cells and unclog pores.

<u>Honey And Cinnamon Scrub</u>

Ingredients:

> 1 tablespoon of raw honey.

> 1 teaspoon of ground cinnamon.

Instructions:

> Pour 1 tsp of honey, add the other tsp of ground cinnamon and mix well.

> Microwave the mixture for 30 seconds before using it then, apply it to your face and let it dry itself for 10-15 minutes.

> Clean your face after it gets all dry.

This mask is good for acne as the honey will help to kill bacteria and the cinnamon will help to dry out pimples. Do not use this mask more than once a week as it can be drying to the skin. You can increase the quantities of ingredients as per your need but avoid making the whole material all at once. Always make a fresh scrub and use it.

So far now, we have studied the benefits and risk factors of several ingredients according to the four acne levels, and how they can be used to treat acne. We have also looked at some recipes that you can use to create your own. Remember to read thoroughly before choosing any of the ingredients because what works for one can might not work for another. Be sure to test any new products on a small area of the skin first to check for allergies. With these tips, now you know exactly what to do and forget about the stress that you are having right now because of your acne.

CHAPTER 7
VITAMINS AND MINERALS

Vitamins are essential nutrients that our body needs to function properly. They play a vital role in various metabolic processes, cell growth, and cell repair, and have an impact on our overall health. Vitamins and minerals are micronutrients that are required by our body to carry out an extension of ordinary functions. In any case, these micronutrients are not created in our bodies and must be obtained by the food we eat. Every living being has distinctive vitamin necessities. For illustration, people have to get Vitamin C from their diets, whereas dogs can produce all the vitamin C that they require.

Vitamins

Vitamins are organic substances that are required in very small amounts for normal growth and metabolism. Vitamins are classified as either water-soluble or fat-soluble. The water-soluble vitamins dissolve in water and are not stored in the body, so they need to be replaced daily. Fat-soluble vitamins are stored in the body's fatty tissue and liver and do not need to be replaced as often.

Water-Soluble Vitamins are substances that can be easily dissolved in water and our body excretes the excess amount of these vitamins through urine.

The human body cannot store these vitamins for a long time, therefore we need a regular dietary intake of these vitamins. The Water-Soluble Vitamins include Vitamin C and all the B-Complex Vitamins (B1, B2, B3, B5, B6, B7, B9, and B12).

Fat-Soluble Vitamins are substances that can be easily dissolved in fats and oils. Unlike Water-Soluble Vitamins, our body can store these vitamins for a long time in the liver and fatty tissues. The Fat-Soluble Vitamins include Vitamins A, D, E, and K.

Vitamin A

Vitamin A is a fat-soluble vitamin and its precursor is (beta-carotene), which is essential for the maintenance of vision, reproduction, mucous membranes, bone and tooth growth, and healthy skin. Its chemical names are " retinol " and "retinal". Vitamin A is also important for the proper functioning of the immune system.

Vitamin A is needed by the both upper and lower layers of skin. It is an antioxidant, which scavenges the harmful free radicals produced by sunlight, pollution, and other environmental factors, prevents them from damaging the skin cells, and also slows down aging. Vitamin A also stimulates the production of collagen and elastin, which helps in keeping the skin firm and elastic.

According to the American Academy of Dermatology (AAD), retinol (retinoid), a topical form of vitamin A, can help treat and prevent inflammatory acne lesions.

How Does Retinol Help In Acne?

Retinol works by binding to retinoic acid receptors (RARs) on the surface of the skin cells. This triggers a chain reaction that leads to the formation of new collagen fibers and increased cell turnover. The new collagen fibers help in filling up the acne scars and the increased cell turnover helps in getting rid of the dead skin cells that can clog pores and lead to breakouts.

It is a type of vitamin A. Retinol is a powerful ingredient that can help to smooth out the skin, promote cell turnover, and diminish the appearance of fine lines and wrinkles.

If you are using a retinol cream, start by using it every other day. Apply a very small amount to the entire face before bedtime. If your skin is not too sensitive, you can increase the frequency every day. Always use sunscreen during the day as retinol can make your skin more sensitive to sunlight.

Side Effects

Yes, retinol can cause side effects like dryness, peeling, and irritation of the skin. Therefore, it is important to start with a lower concentration and gradually increase it as your skin gets used to it. It is also important to use sunscreen while using retinol as it can make your skin more sensitive to sunlight.

The recommended dietary allowance (RDA) for vitamin A is 900 micrograms/day for men and 700 micrograms/day for women. Health experts recommend 5,000 IU of vitamin A per day.

There is an old saying " Excess of everything is bad", taking too much vitamin A can cause some worse effects too. Hypervitaminosis A is a rare but serious condition that can occur when you take more than the recommended amount of vitamin A. Symptoms of hypervitaminosis A include headaches, dry skin, joint pain, and vomiting. In severe cases, it can lead to liver damage and death.

Vitamin A is found in animal products like milk, eggs, cheese, liver, and fish oil. Plant-based foods that are rich in vitamin A include carrots, sweet potatoes, spinach, kale, and broccoli.

Vitamin D

Vitamin D is a fat-soluble vitamin that is synthesized in the body when our skin is exposed to sunlight. It is also known as the "sunshine vitamin". Chemically it is known as " ergocalciferol " and " cholecalciferol ". Individuals with vitamin D deficiencies are more vulnerable to acne. Vitamin D is important for the absorption of calcium and phosphorus, which are needed for the development and maintenance of strong bones and teeth. Vitamin D is also known to boost the immune system and has anti-inflammatory properties.

A study published in the Journal of Drugs in Dermatology found that a vitamin D3 cream was effective in the treatment of mild to moderate acne. The study found that the cream reduced the number of acne lesions and also improved the appearance of the skin.

Vitamin D levels were associated with increased severity of acne. People who had nodulocystic acne had the lowest levels of vitamin D. It is not a listed risk factor for acne but according to recent searches, vitamin D deficiency leads to acne, and raising the levels of vitamin D in your body through diet or supplements end up benefiting acne-prone skins.

In another study, individuals with acne experienced altogether progressed symptoms when they took oral vitamin D supplements.

The Institute of Medicine (IOM) recommends a daily intake of 600 IU (15 micrograms) of vitamin D for adults. However, some health experts recommend a daily intake of 1000-2000 IU (25-50 micrograms) that has the lowest levels of vitamin D.

Vitamin D is an essential fat-soluble vitamin, there are different ways of getting vitamin D and using the source properly:

➢ **Directly from the sun** - In case you are vitamin D deficient, sitting in the sun would not help you in setting your acne. Spend 10-15 minutes in the sun 2-3 times a week. Make sure that your skin is not covered with sunscreen as it will block the synthesis of vitamin D. Also, getting vitamin D directly from the sun is not a recommended source according to experts. Because prolonged exposure to sunshine without applying sunscreen can increase your risk of getting skin cancer.

➢ **Food sources** - Foods that are rich in vitamin D include fatty fish like salmon, mackerel, and tuna. You can also get it from egg yolks, cheese, and beef liver. Be careful while increasing the levels of vitamin D in your diet because taking excess vitamin D can create toxicity in your body which can lead to "hypercalcemia". This is a condition where there is an abnormally high level of calcium in the blood.

➢ **Supplements** - If you are not getting enough vitamin D from your diet or from the sun, you can consider taking supplements for correcting your deficiency and acne. The most recommended vitamin D supplements are (Vitamin D3 supplements), which are available over the counter. Additionally, taking vitamin D through supplements is believed as the best source to help acne. Vitamin D supplements result in best when taken with the diet.

➤ **Topical application** - There are different topical products available in the market that contain vitamin D. You can apply it directly to your acne-prone skin. The topical application of vitamin D has been proven to be an effective way to induce vitamin D levels with fewer side effects than oral supplements.

Vitamin E

Vitamin E is also a fat-soluble vitamin that has antioxidant and anti-inflammatory properties. It works with vitamin C to strengthen cell walls. Its chemical name is "tocopherol" and "tocotrienol" because it is made up of four tocopherol proteins and four tocotrienol proteins which are fat-soluble compounds. Vitamin E prevents oxidative stress by scavenging harmful ROS. It also helps in membrane stabilization by reducing the oxidation of lipids. There are also some other major functions of vitamin E including protection against various diseases, inhibition of platelet coagulation, a biocompatible modifier of biomaterials, and medical devices.

Vitamin E deficiency causes dry skin, which ultimately causes acne. Vitamin E is also famous as " the vitamin of beauty" because it nourishes the skin and makes it healthy. Healthy skin is the only key to avoiding acne. Your skin can get effortlessly bothered and inflamed when it is dry. Keeping it moisturized is critical and with vitamin E, a defensive oil boundary is formed which locks the moisture inside the skin. Another incredible property is that it may also progress the bloodstream, which in turn progresses the scalp and hair health.

Vitamin E is available in the form of capsules, which can be taken orally. The other way is to directly apply it to your skin. Vitamin E oil is retained in the skin rapidly since it is a fat-soluble vitamin. This leads to quicker recuperating of acne and acne scars. It controls the formation of collagen and elastin within the skin. The collagen fortifies the skin and may offer assistance with the skin's flexibility and hydration. It can decrease skin wrinkles and dryness as well.

Whatever the way you are using, just keep an eye on the dosage because taking an excessive amount of vitamin E supplements can lead to "hypervitaminosis E" which is a condition where there is an abnormally high level of vitamin E in the body. The common symptoms of hypervitaminosis E include nausea, abdominal pain, weakness, fatigue, and diarrhea.

Some of the time it is best to utilize the vitamin E oil by itself. Other times it is nice to blend it with other items, such as night cream or lotion. The primary step to battling acne is to know your skin sort and be mindful of your body changes. That way your skin will be thankful to you.

Applying it directly to your skin can be done with a cotton swab. Just put some vitamin E cream, oil, lotion, and whatever form of product you are using on the cotton swab and apply it to your skin in a circular motion. You can also mix the capsules with your other night creams or lotion and apply them before going to bed. Do not scrub so much and harshly, leave it wet and let the skin absorb and get dry itself.

Vitamin E has no Recommended Dietary Allowance (RDA) but the American Dietetic Association (ADA) suggests a daily intake of 15 mg. The Linus Pauling Institute at Oregon State University also recommends the same dosage. You can get your recommended daily value from dietary sources like nuts, seeds, vegetable oils, leafy greens, and fortified cereals. You can also take supplements but it is always suggested to first increase your intake from dietary sources. The reason is that people who consume a lot of vitamin E from dietary sources have a lower risk of prostate cancer as compared to those who take supplements.

Vitamin E supplementation has been studied for a long time for its potential role in acne vulgaris treatment. A four-week study was conducted on 35 patients with mild to moderate acne. The participants were asked to apply a lotion containing 0.5% vitamin E and 2% vitamin C twice daily. The results of the study showed that there was a significant reduction in both inflammatory and non-inflammatory acne lesions.

Vitamin E supplements are available in different forms like capsules, tablets, and liquids. You can also find natural and synthetic forms of vitamin E supplements. The natural form is labeled as d-alpha-tocopherol while the synthetic form is labeled as dl-alpha-tocopherol. Both natural and synthetic forms are equally effective but it is always better to go with the natural form.

Minerals

Minerals are inorganic substances that are required by our bodies to carry out various functions. Unlike vitamins, minerals cannot be synthesized by our body and must be obtained through our diet. Minerals are classified as either major minerals or trace minerals. Major minerals are required in large amounts by our body, whereas trace minerals are required in very small amounts.

Major minerals are inorganic substances that are required in large amounts by our bodies for various functions. The major minerals include calcium, phosphorus, magnesium, sodium, potassium, chloride, and sulfur.

Trace Minerals are inorganic substances that are required in very small amounts by our body for various functions. The trace minerals include iron, copper, iodine, zinc, selenium, manganese, chromium, and molybdenum.

Zinc

Zinc is a mineral that is required in very small amounts by our bodies for various functions. It is classified as a trace mineral. Zinc plays a fundamental part in the catalysis of over 100 metabolic and enzymatic exercises within the body, and it is necessary for homeostasis and adjustment within the system. Furthermore, zinc plays an important role in the immune system, DNA synthesis, and cell growth. It is also involved in the metabolism of carbohydrates, proteins, and fats.

Zinc is one of the foremost broadly considered minerals for skin break out treatment. Concurring with Dermatology Investigate and Practice, both natural and salt forms of zinc can resolve a wide run of skin afflictions. The antioxidant effect on aggravation and bacteria-fighting properties are the two essential ways that zinc can diminish the event of acne and breakouts.

Antioxidant Effect - A large portion of the hurt that prompts skin aggravation and breakouts is oxidative stress. This kind of stress happens when there's an unequal number of electrons in a particle. This can make the particle unstable, which makes it more inclined to respond to different particles and produce free radicals.

Zinc is a natural DHT- blocker which lowers the level of sebum. Zinc can help diminish the severity of acne by blocking the conversion of testosterone to DHT. DHT is a hormone that is known to aggravate acne. In the absence of zinc, normal apoptosis fails to occur, cells overgrow which causes an unnatural build-up of dying cells.

The utilization of topical or dietary zinc could be a common treatment for pubescent acne(acne vulgaris). Zinc is known for its anti-inflammatory, antibacterial, and sebum-reducing properties. When zinc is combined with alpha and beta hydroxy acids, it can be an extremely successful acne-fighting duo. Because it swamps off the remaining cells from the dried sebum and reduces excessively active sebaceous glands.

Antibacterial Effect - The second way that zinc can diminish the event of acne and breakouts is by battling bacteria. Zinc is naturally antimicrobial and can steadily murder-off acne-causing bacteria with less potential impact. As we have already discussed in chapter 1 that one of the principal reasons that skin break out creates an excess of Propionibacterium acnes (P. acnes) bacteria on the skin. This kind of bacteria feeds off of sebum, when there is an excess of sebum on the skin, it can create an ideal environment for bacteria to grow.

A 2014 study investigates the blood levels of zinc, vitamin A, and vitamin E in people with and without acne. The researchers found that the levels of all of these vitamins and minerals were significantly lower in people with acne.

Zinc also helps in the conversion of proteins into vitamin A which is involved in the cell reproduction process. When zinc converts vitamin A into retinol-A they kill acne-causing bacteria. Zinc is also known to possess wound-healing properties and can help in the healing of acne scars.

The Recommended Dietary Allowance (RDA) is 8-11mg/day for adult females and 11-14 mg/day for adult males. Zinc can be found in a variety of foods like oysters, crab, lobster, fortified cereals, red meat, poultry, beans, nuts, whole grains, and dairy products.

Oysters are by far the best source of zinc providing 74 mg per 100g, crab and lobster provide 3-6mg/100g. Fortified breakfast cereals provide around 25% of the RDA. Red meat, poultry, beans, nuts, whole grains, and dairy products provide around 5-10% of the RDA.

Zinc Supplements

Zinc supplements are available in a variety of forms like tablets, capsules, liquids, and lozenges. Zinc supplements are generally safe when taken at the recommended doses. The most common side effects are gastrointestinal problems like nausea, vomiting, and diarrhea. Taking zinc on an empty stomach can increase the risk of these side effects.

Zinc supplements can interact with a variety of medications like antibiotics, bisphosphonates, penicillamine, and quinolone antibiotics. Zinc can also reduce the absorption of copper which can lead to copper deficiency. People with Wilson's disease should avoid zinc supplements as they can worsen their condition.

Pregnant women and young children should avoid taking zinc supplements as they can be at risk of zinc toxicity. Zinc supplements should be taken with caution in people with kidney disease as they may be at risk of zinc toxicity.

Bioavailability

Zinc sulfate is the most bioavailable form of zinc supplement. However, it is also the most likely to cause side effects like nausea and vomiting. Zinc gluconate is the next most bioavailable form of zinc supplement. It is less likely to cause side effects than zinc sulfate but more expensive.

Zinc oxide is a popular ingredient in sunscreen and diaper rash cream. It is also used as an astringent and antiseptic. Zinc oxide is a white powder that is insoluble in water. It is used in a variety of products because it has the ability to reflect light and absorb ultraviolet (UV) light.

Selenium

Selenium is a trace element that is essential for human health. Selenium helps to improve the immune system, thyroid function, and fertility. Selenium deficiency is rare but can happen in people with diets that lack selenium-rich foods or in people with gastrointestinal disorders like Crohn's disease.

In the case of acne taking, selenium alone will not gonna work. For treating acne selenium has to work synergistically with vitamin E and zinc. Selenium helps in increasing the overall antioxidant level of the body which as a result decreases the inflammation that contributes to acne. It also helps to decrease inflammatory acne directly.

Selenium also protects us from heavy metals like mercury and arsenic. Mercury is often found in sea foods and arsenic is found in vegetables. These heavy metals harm our body very badly by increasing the levels of inflammation in the body and making our body insulin resistant which results in acne.

Another most loved attribute of selenium is that it protects our body from UV damage by making our skin more grounded and more sun resistant. People who eat enough levels of selenium minimize their risk of getting skin cancer even if they get exposed to the sun more often.

The most important function of selenium is glutathione peroxidase production. Glutathione peroxidase is an enzyme that scavenges for hydrogen peroxide and other reactive oxygen species (ROS). These reactive oxygen species are known for triggering and worsening the effects of acne.

The Recommended Dietary Allowance (RDA) for selenium is 55 mcg/day for adults. Pregnant and lactating women need 60 mcg/day and 70 mcg/day, respectively. The Upper Limit (UL) for selenium is 400 mcg/day for adults.

The best food sources of selenium are Brazil nuts, tuna, shrimp, salmon, whole wheat bread, and brown rice. One Brazil nut can provide the RDA for selenium. Tuna, shrimp, and salmon provide around 50% of the RDA for selenium.

Likewise, other minerals and selenium supplements are also available in the forms of tablets, capsules, and liquid. The most popular selenium supplement is SelenoExcell, which is a high-selenium yeast supplement, which essentially decreases the biomarkers for oxidative stress, which are measures of sound maturing and decreased chance for unremitting sickness and certain cancers.

Selenium toxicity is very rare and only happens in people who work with selenium-containing chemicals or have accidents involving selenium. Symptoms of selenium toxicity include garlic breath, nausea, vomiting, upset stomach, fatigue, irritability, hair loss, and brittle nails.

CHAPTER 8
TREATMENTS

One thing we already know is that most people will get acne at some time during their lives. One can develop acne at any level of his/her life. Even babies can develop acne, but it is most prevalent in teenagers. Acne vulgaris, which is the most common form of acne, affects people during their teenage years and early twenties. In some people, however, the condition may persist in adulthood. You should consult a doctor if your baby develops acne that does not clear up on its own within three months.

This chapter will discuss some of the most popular treatments and remedies for acne. It is important to remember that these remedies may not work for everyone. Always speak to a doctor before trying any new treatment, especially if you have a history of skin conditions.

Treatments For Acne

Severe acne can be treated with a few medical procedures, though they are less common than medication. Most of the time, these procedures can be done in your doctor's office. They might hurt and, in some cases, leave scars. They are also not always covered by health insurance plans. Before scheduling these procedures, check to see if they are covered by your insurance.

Laser Therapy

It may appear that lasers and other light therapies are the best way to treat acne. To get rid of the acne, simply shine a light. Even in the skilled hands of a dermatologist, using them is actually a little more involved and the outcomes are less predictable. Nonetheless, these treatments might be a good addition to an acne treatment plan.

Acne can benefit greatly from these treatments. When laser therapy was added to a treatment plan for severe acne cysts, some patients saw relief for years. Laser therapy uses a focused beam of light to kill the bacteria that cause acne. It can also help to reduce the inflammation and redness associated with acne.

Things To Know About Laser Therapy For Acne

Before you make laser therapy your go-to option, you need to know that scars can be less noticeable with laser treatment, but they cannot be removed. When you have laser scar treatment, one scar is replaced with another that is less obvious.

You may not get the results of your desire if the person performing your laser therapy lacks medical expertise. Moreover, it can be very risky. Prior to beginning any laser treatment, a medical consultation is essential. Walk away from a person who promises to treat your scar before offering a medical consultation.

A serious burn or skin discoloration could result from using a laser. You will need to protect your skin from the sun while it heals from laser treatment. You might get another scar if the sun hits your treated skin with harmful rays.

A dermatologist might plan a series of laser treatments for a patient to get the best possible results that last for a long time. When employing a type of laser known as a non-ablative laser, this is frequently required. With this laser, you won't have to take any time off, but you might need a few treatments to get the results you want.

Laser and light therapies typically produce lasting results. However, patients frequently require follow-up treatments once or twice a year to maintain results.

Types Of Laser And Lights

Acne nodules, blackheads, whiteheads, and pimples can all be treated with laser or light therapy alone. Acne is treated with a variety of lasers and light therapies as a result. What the various types of lasers and lights can and cannot treat is explained in the following.

Red + Blue light Devices - One of the most common types of laser and light therapy for acne is a device that emits both red and blue light. These devices are available without a prescription, which means you can use them at home. These devices, which are known as visible light because you can see the colors, can treat pimples. Acne nodules, blackheads, whiteheads, and acne cysts cannot be removed with visible light.

Infrared light Devices - Acne can be treated with an infrared device, which is also available without a prescription. It is invisible to the eye and can penetrate deep into the skin. As a result, it is ideal for treating acne nodules and cysts. These devices are frequently used in spas and salons as well.

A dermatologist in their office frequently uses light and laser therapy to treat acne. The most sophisticated devices are available only in a doctor's office.

These are FDA-cleared for the treatment of acne and can be very successful. A device that emits both red and blue light, for example, may be used in a doctor's office. IPL, which is short for intense pulsed light, can be used as well. This device emits a broad spectrum of light that can treat acne and acne scars.

Photodynamic Therapy (PDT)

This is a treatment that can also be done in a doctor's office. First, a chemical is applied to the skin. This chemical makes the skin more sensitive to light. The solution needs to remain on the skin for at least 15 minutes to three hours. A dermatologist then treats the skin with a light or laser device. As a result, the pimples are less likely to return.

Photopneumatic Therapy (PPT)

An intense pulsed light (IPL) laser and a gentle vacuum are used in this treatment. It clears clogged pores by removing excess oil and dead skin cells. Blackheads, whiteheads, and some pimples can all be treated with this FDA-approved treatment. It is unable to treat acne cysts or nodules. A machine that uses suction is first placed on the skin.

The suction opens up the pores and helps to remove the sebum, which is the oil that clogs the pores and causes acne. The device is then turned off, and a light or laser device is used to kill the bacteria that cause acne.

Drainage and Extraction

A small, blunt-tipped instrument is used to break up the blackheads and whiteheads. The contents of the pimple are then removed with gentle suction. This is an effective way to treat acne but can only be done once every four to six weeks.

A dermatological procedure known as acne extraction is used to get rid of common forms of acne, such as blackheads and whiteheads. A dermatologist will use a sterile, specialized instrument known as a comedone extractor to physically remove the contents of blocked pores during an acne extraction procedure. The dermatologist may use an exfoliant to get rid of extra skin cells before extracting the contents of your acne. After that, they may use alcohol to prepare the targeted areas to prevent bacteria from getting onto your skin during the extraction process.

The fact that acne extraction yields immediate results is one of its greatest advantages. Acne extraction eliminates cystic acne in a single procedure, in contrast to acne creams, gels, and cleansers, which can take weeks to begin working. Another advantage of acne extraction is that it can treat comedones that are large or hard to get rid of with medication.

Acne can be a difficult thing to deal with, but there are treatments available that can help. Although there are numerous advantages to acne extraction, it is not always the most effective treatment for acne. After an extraction, you may need to take medication to prevent infection and inflammation to protect your skin.

Hormonal Therapies

Acne sufferers who have hormonal conditions like polycystic ovary syndrome or when their acne flares up around their periods may benefit from hormonal treatments. Even if you are not sexually active, a doctor may recommend the combined oral contraceptive pill to you if you do not already use it.

This combination pill often helps women with acne, but it may take up to a year for the full effects to show. Acne treatment may include hormone therapy. The body's various organs, including the skin, are controlled by hormones, which are chemicals that circulate in the blood.

Co-Cyprindiol Treatment

Co-cyprindiol is a hormonal treatment for acne that does not respond to antibiotics and is more severe. It aids in the reduction of sebum production. It is likely that you will need to use co-cyprindiol for anywhere from two to six months before your acne significantly improves.

Women who take co-cyprindiol run a small chance of developing breast cancer in later life.

It is a type of medication that is taken as a pill and has both an anti-androgen (testosterone-blocking) and an estrogen effect. This makes it useful in treating acne in women who do not respond to other treatments such as antibiotics or the combined oral contraceptive pill.

Additionally, there is a very small chance that co-cyprindiol will cause a blood clot. In any given year, the risk is estimated to be around 1 in 2,500. Co-cyprindiol should not be taken if you are pregnant or breastfeeding. Before treatment can begin, women may be required to have a pregnancy test.

Spironolactone Hormonal Therapy

This medication is prescribed by doctors to treat high blood pressure. Additionally, it is prescribed for individuals with excessive fluid retention. It has been prescribed by dermatologists for many years to treat women's acne and excessive hair growth.

It can effectively treat tender, deep-seated acne on the lower face, jawline, or neck when other acne treatments fail. Due to its negative effects, men's acne treatment with spironolactone is not recommended. Men who take this acne medication have developed breasts.

Spironolactone is generally regarded as safe for women in good health. The pill and spironolactone can both improve effectiveness. Another benefit comes from this combination. Spironolactone should only be taken with birth control. Spironolactone can cause serious birth defects in unborn babies if you become pregnant while taking it.

It is also possible to prescribe spironolactone without a pill. The pill may not be an option for you if you are 35 or older, and only spironolactone may be prescribed. When you have a medical condition that makes it unsafe to take the pill, such as having had a blood clot or stroke, it is also recommended to take spironolactone without the pill.

Spironolactone can be quite effective when taken by itself. Researchers examined the medical records of 85 women who took spironolactone and discovered that one-third of the women experienced complete acne clearing and one-third experienced significantly less acne. Only 7% reported no change.

Side effects of spironolactone include irregular periods, breast tenderness, headaches, and dizziness. If you experience any of these side effects, contact your doctor. Spironolactone should not be taken during pregnancy as it can cause birth defects.

Steroids Injections

Most of the time, steroid injections are used to treat acne that causes painful lumps under the skin (nodules and cysts). It can take weeks for these conditions to go away on their own. Steroid injections can reduce pain, flatten lumps, and clear skin in as little as a few days.

Despite its effectiveness, this medication can cause the following side effects: Skin tone that becomes lighter than usual and thinning of the skin. Steroid injections are usually used as a temporary or occasional treatment for stubborn cysts and nodules. Because of the potential side effects and the need for frequent doctor visits, they are not used to treat widespread acne.

Acne gets worse when it develops scars. And to treat scars, sometimes scars are injected with various substances such as collagen, fat, or a variety of synthetic materials. These substances may raise the scarred area to make it level with the rest of the skin. Fillers such as collagen, hyaluronic acid, and polymethylmethacrylate injections are temporary and must be repeated periodically. Some of the other injections are permanent.

Overall, hormonal therapies are a safe and effective way of treating acne in any age group. It might be an option for people who want to get rid of their acne as soon as possible and want quick results. However, before attempting any treatment, you should be aware that there are some risk factors associated with each method. You are not alone in this battle against acne; all you have to do is accept your skin's current state and begin the process of fixing it.

Non- Pharmaceutical Treatments

Chemical Peels And Microdermabrasion

These are the two other possible treatments for acne. A chemical peel is a skin-resurfacing procedure in which a chemical solution is applied to the skin to remove the top layers. The strength of the peel will determine how many layers of skin are removed. A light chemical peel can be done in an office visit and will remove the outermost layer of skin. A deeper peel may require sedation and can remove layers of skin from the face, neck, chest, or hands.

When you shed the top layer of your skin, living skin cells will be told to multiply and move to the surface. This sends a signal to your body to produce more collagen, which will make your skin more elastic. The natural production of hyaluronic acid is also boosted by the reaction.

Your skin will start to look and feel younger as a result.

Your skincare products will perform better after a chemical peel. Your skin no longer has dead skin cells on its surface. Your products will have an easier time getting under the skin and starting to work as a result of this.

You can choose from mild to deep chemical peels among three main categories. Different skin conditions can be treated with each formula. A deep peel, on the other hand, is the best option for wrinkles and deep scars. A single deep chemical peel typically yields results after just one session, in contrast to other peels, which may necessitate multiple treatments. However, a deep peel will take longer to heal, anywhere from six to twelve months.

Older customers are fans of deep peels. These peels have the potential to lessen the appearance of wrinkles around the mouth, eyes, and forehead. A medium peel is also effective for lines with moderate width.

Microdermabrasion uses a device that blows fine crystals across the skin to remove the outermost layer of dead skin cells. It can be easily performed in an office visit and does not require anesthesia. While treating acne, microdermabrasion can also address wrinkle lines, frown lines, age spots, and other skin abnormalities, in addition to assisting you in achieving a clearer complexion.

Because the treatment only takes up to 60 minutes, microdermabrasion is frequently referred to as a "lunchtime" procedure. Additionally, there is no discomfort or downtime, so you can resume your normal activities almost immediately.

When you have active acne, microdermabrasion can break up those spots, making your acne worse, extending your healing time, and increasing your risk of infection. Because microdermabrasion can put some stress on the cells in your skin, your acne might look worse for a while before getting better. If you are patient, you will achieve your goals.

Both chemical peels and microdermabrasion can help to improve the appearance of acne scars. However, neither procedure will get rid of them completely. If you have tried self-care measures without success, make an appointment to see a dermatologist.

CHAPTER 9

HOW TO CHOOSE MEDICATION

You have worked hard to get rid of your acne, and now you feel like you're stuck. You are unsure whether to break down and schedule an appointment with a dermatologist or stick with what you are doing. You will learn how to choose the right medication and when to do so in this chapter, which will assist you in clearing up your confusion.

Do Not Mix It With Other Disease

Every person has experienced a pimple at some point in their lives. People do not like them, but annoyance and shame are typically the most serious issues that come from acne.

However, there are times when what we mistake for a typical zit may actually be another skin condition that calls for more than just a cream from the drugstore.

Acne diagnosis is another crucial step. You should see a dermatologist as soon as possible if you notice any changes to your skin because you might confuse them with other skin issues. Your skin problem can be easily identified by a dermatologist, who can then begin treatment.

Other Diseases Like Acne

Folliculitis

It is a skin condition that can easily get confused with acne. It occurs when the hair follicle is infected with yeast or bacteria, it swells up, causing these small bumps to appear. These bumps can occur anywhere on your body that has hair, but the neck, legs, armpits, and buttocks are the most common locations. These minuscule clusters of blisters may also be referred to as hot tub rash, barber's itch, or razor bumps.

With basic self-care, mild cases usually go away in a few days. Folliculitis can be caused by heat and sweat, so take a shower after working out hard. You will need the assistance of your doctor if it continues to occur or lingers. A topical antibiotic or anti-yeast treatment may be tried from time to time in addition to oral antibiotics.

Rosacea

It also gets often mistaken for acne or an allergy. Redness on the cheeks and nose is a common symptom of this condition, but it can also be accompanied by red bumps. It usually comes from families. Stress, alcohol, smoking, heat, sun, and other factors can all contribute to outbreaks.

Topical creams that sometimes contain low-dose antibiotics are some of the treatments. Sunlight can exacerbate rosacea, so if you are prone to it, always wear sunscreen when outside.

Staph

Staph bacteria can occasionally cause large, painful bumps that look like acne. Staphylococcus aureus, a type of bacteria, is all around us at all times: on our bodies, in our noses, on surfaces and the ground, and on our skin

The most common type of staph infection is a blemish on the skin that is inflamed. Antibiotics are usually sufficient to treat these minor infections. The infections become significantly more severe if they enter the bloodstream, bones, joints, or organs.

Consult your doctor if a blemish hurts or does not go away. Similar to how you can avoid the common cold, flu, and other illnesses, you can avoid these staph infections: Avoid touching your face and wash your hands frequently.

Keratosis Pilaris

It is a very common genetic skin condition that can be very hard to treat and looks like acne. The appearance and location of the bumps are the main distinctions between keratosis pilaris and acne. Dry, rough bumps appear on the sides of the upper arms, face, thighs, and buttocks of people with this condition. On the other hand, acne affects your back, chest, and face.

Due to their white filling, these bumps can resemble acne pustules and are caused by an excess of a protein known as the keratin in the hair follicle openings. However, Waibel explains that sebum, an oily substance, is what fills acne spots.

Shainhouse explains that moisturizers and topical exfoliators, such as alpha and beta hydroxy acids (like salicylic, lactic, or glycolic acids), can be used to treat keratosis pilaris, which does tend to get better with age. However, if those do not assist, it is suggested to discuss a prescription retinoid with your physician.

Periorificial dermatitis

It is also an acne-like eruption that is more likely to develop in women and children, and presents with persistent pink bumps around the facial openings (eyes, nose, and mouth). If periorificial dermatitis is not treated properly, this condition can last for months or even years.

If you do have this condition, your doctor will give you antibiotic creams and tablets and anti-inflammatory drugs to get rid of the breakout. However, be ready to wait at least a month or longer for it to completely clear.

Skin cancer

Small, pearly bumps that can be pink, red, blue, brown, or black can be the beginning of skin cancer. Suspect pink growths also have raised edges and a lower area in the middle. This is the stage where you can confuse it with acne.

Skin cancer may also be present in open wounds that do not heal or heal only to return. Consult your physician if you notice any of these bumps or lesions. Do not dismiss them as merely cosmetic. If caught early, skin cancer can be easily treated; however, if it is not caught before it spreads, it can be fatal.

According to Dr. Fox, it is essential to keep in mind that not all red bumps on your skin are caused by acne. Even if a flaw is causing you pain, do not ignore it too quickly. Even if it's a common pimple, there are treatments for it if it is causing you physical or emotional pain.

Why Acne Should Be Treated Early

Numerous negative effects on life can result from acne. It may result in physical, emotional, and scarring pain. Acne can also cause depression and social anxiety. To avoid these negative outcomes, prompt treatment is essential.

You might decide to let the acne go away on its own if your teen or preteen has it. However, treating acne when it first appears may be the most effective approach.

Some of the scientifically supported reasons which suggest that early treatment is your best option are:

> **Get treatment results faster** - Whether you're treating moderate or severe acne, acne treatment takes time. However, clearing a few pimples takes less time and effort than clearing a variety of breakouts, including blackheads, whiteheads, and deep-seated acne cysts.

> **Reduce wounds** - Acne scarring can be avoided by treating it early. In general, scarring is more likely to occur when acne is severe. Mild acne can leave scars when picked up, whereas severe acne is more likely to leave scars. If an individual treats their acne at the first sign of it, it may also prevent them from picking at it regularly, preventing acne scarring.

> **When acne is gone, stop spots from coming back** - When an acne nodule, cyst, or pimple clears, a dark spot may appear for anyone with skin that is medium to darkly pigmented. This is known as post-inflammatory hyperpigmentation (PIH) by dermatologists. Where acne used to be, people with light skin may see a red spot.

These areas may persist for months. Many people think that having these lingering spots is worse than having acne. Acne can start in childhood. Acne sufferers aged 7 to 12 are now seen by dermatologists. Acne can be prevented from coming back by treating it early and keeping it under control. In today's world, that could amount to a significant number of years without acne. Acne affects many people in their 20s. Acne can last well into one's 30s, 40s, or even 50s or 60s for some adults.

➢ **Avoid emotional turmoil** - Acne can result in more than just pimples. Acne can also have a negative psychological impact, according to research. Acne, according to many, had a negative impact on their self-esteem. Acne sufferers may withdraw from their social circle. It does not appear to matter how severe the acne is. Whether you have mild or severe acne, it can hurt your relationships and self-esteem. Acne was found to be linked to depression and suicidal ideation in a large study. These feelings can be alleviated by treating acne, according to other studies.

When You Need Prescription Treatment

How can you tell when it is time to switch to a prescription acne treatment? The five warning signs and indications that it is time to take prescription acne medication are as follows:

OTC Products Does Not Work

When you start getting acne, it's natural to want to buy some over-the-counter acne treatments. Additionally, for some individuals, many of these over-the-counter products are extremely effective.

But not all over-the-counter treatments work. If you have been using over-the-counter acne products on a regular basis for several months and your acne has not improved, it may be time to switch to stronger products.

Your Acne Gets Severe or Inflamed

If your acne has reached the severity level and you are just sticking to over-the-counter medications what you need to know is that they are best for mild breakouts only. They just would not work for severe acne.

Because moderate to severe inflammatory acne is difficult to treat, working with an experienced dermatologist to develop a treatment plan will significantly improve your outcomes.

You Are Developing Acne Scars

If your acne is causing scars or you are aware that your skin is particularly prone to scarring, you should get a prescription medication as soon as possible. Unlike permanent acne scars, acne breakouts are much simpler to treat.

Make an appointment with the dermatologist right away. Acne will cause less long-term damage to your skin if you begin taking a prescription medication as soon as possible.

What about the scars you already have from acne? Numerous acne scar treatments yield impressive outcomes. After your acne is under control and your skin is generally clear, scar treatment procedures are performed.

Large Areas Get Affected

Acne does not just affect the face; you're breaking out over large areas of your body as well. It likes to appear anywhere, including on your bum, chest, and shoulders.

Widespread acne is typically more difficult to treat, and body acne tends to be particularly stubborn. The best course of action, in this case, is a prescription drug.

You Have No Idea What to Do Next

Attempting to treat acne on your own can be completely overwhelming. Call your dermatologist if you are not sure what to do about your acne or just need some help coming up with a treatment plan. This is especially true if you are depressed about your skin or think your acne is making your life harder. Prescription acne medications should be prescribed by a doctor in these situations.

Keep in mind that it is better to get the right medication from a doctor than to waste time and money on over-the-counter products that just do not work for you. Therefore, even though scheduling an appointment with a dermatologist may appear to be a hassle, it will ultimately be worth it.

We hope that now you have learned about when it's time to switch to prescription acne medication and a dermatologist for help. You will be the first dermatologist you meet. Before considering acne, take note of every minute change to your skin; even if it's not acne, you never know what else it could be. A red, itchy rash could be a sign of infections or allergies, and a red "butterfly" rash on your face could be lupus. A yellow hue could be an indication of liver disease. Additionally, dark or unusual moles may be a sign of skin cancer. If you notice anything out of the ordinary with your skin, check with your doctor.

CHAPTER 10

HOW TO MAINTAIN

The saying goes, "beauty is only skin deep; "What matters is what's on the "inside."Although our skin serves as the first line of defense against the outside world, our internal organs are certainly important. Additionally, your skin can provide crucial health-related information. Learn how to take care of your skin so that it can continue to take good care of you.

We already know that the skin is the largest organ in the human body, and being so entrusted with so much responsibility is no accident. The importance of the skin cannot be overstated, whether it is maintaining the moisture balance of the circulatory system. Despite the fact that almost everything you do has an impact on your skin, many people do not properly care for their skin.

There are a few reasons why we should not skip our regular skincare routines and why we should keep our skin healthy. These reasons are explained as follows:

More Rapid Healing

Your skin will be damaged and exposed to the elements unless you intend to live in a bubble for the rest of your life. You will at some point cause damage to your skin, whether it be from scraping your shin while playing with your child or cutting your finger while cooking in the kitchen. Because healthy skin is better able to regenerate and heal itself, you can heal more quickly and are less likely to catch an infection. Skin is less prone to minor abrasions when it is treated with topical products that improve barrier protection. That is why you need to take care of your skin so that it will heal fast.

To Give The Comfort

To put it simply, comfortable skin is healthy skin. The majority of us have experienced dry, dehydrated skin at some point. So we are aware of the potential discomfort. Our skin is less prone to damage and irritation when it is properly cleansed, moisturized, and nourished.

Your Overall Appearance

To be honest, healthy skin looks better than unhealthy skin. Taking care of your skin can help you look younger and younger-looking at the same time. It is not a crime to want to look good, and taking care of your skin is a great way to achieve that goal.

Preventing Disease

What we understood yet is that the primary barrier between your vital organs and the outside world is your skin. As a result, it prevents diseases, germs, and other harmful substances from entering your body and causing harm. Skin that is healthy is better able to protect you from things that would otherwise make you sick.

Prevention is Better Than Treatment

It is true that prevention is preferable to treatment, particularly when it comes to skincare. It's possible that taking better care of your skin will help you save money in the long run on costly skin repairs. Not only will paying attention to your skin now help you look better, but it will also keep you from having to worry about things like acne scars, deep wrinkles, advanced skin aging, skin discoloration, and even skin cancer.

Problems with the skin that are caused by neglect or a lack of skin care may require more time—and money! than simply adhering to a daily skincare regimen.

Best Skincare Routine For Acne-Prone Skins

Isn't it unfair that some people have flawless skin all the time? They may be on a restricted diet or have won the genetic lottery. Or maybe they have a strict skincare routine that makes their skin smooth, free of pores, and free of blemishes.

It is important to remember that we all have different skin, so do not get discouraged. Some individuals might have normal skin that is neither oily nor dry. Some people have oily skin that is prone to breakouts and clogged pores. Additionally, there are those who require intense hydration and have dry skin.

Let's have a quick look at the best recommended and tested healthy skincare routine for acne-prone skins. If you follow this regime we promise your skin will thank you for this.

Step 1- Cleanse

Use a mild, pH-balanced cleanser to wash your face one to two times per day. Skin barrier disruption caused by harsh cleansers leads to more problems than they solve. If you've been using sunscreen or makeup, do not forget to wash twice!

Importance of this step: Surfactants, detergents that work to remove unwanted substances and particles from the skin's outermost layer, are found in facial cleansers. Depending on the skincare product you use, these surfactants work by attracting oil, makeup, dirt, and debris so that they can be rinsed away more easily.

Which cleansers you can use: A number of cleansers include additional ingredients to address common skin issues like acne. *Acne cleansers,* some acne-prone skin cleansers simply do not contain any oils or ingredients that are irritating. However, other treatments, such as those for acne at home, use ingredients like salicylic acid or benzoyl peroxide to make your skin look better.

Cleansers that exfoliate, and facial cleansers may contain tiny particles to mechanically remove dead skin cells. These are best used once or twice a week, but you should not use them too much because they could dry out your skin

Step 2 - Moisturizer

Even if your skin is oily, this step is a must for healthy skin and cannot be skipped. Finding one that works well for you is the hard part. Moisturize your skin for around 2 to 3 minutes. When you apply it after washing your face, it helps your skin retain the water it needs.

Importance of this step: Your body produces more oil when your skin becomes dry. Your pores may become clogged by the additional oil, resulting in additional breakouts. You can keep your skin from becoming dry and irritated with the right moisturizer.

Right moisturizer for acne: Look for one of the following descriptions on the container of a moisturizer to ensure that it does not cause breakouts: Free of oil, non-comedogenic, and would not clog pores.

Step 3 - SPF

UV rays can aggravate acne and leave scars, redness, and post-acne marks. Therefore, especially if you are going to be out in the sun, do not forget to apply SPF in the morning. When the sun's rays are at their strongest, avoid the area between 10 a.m. and 4 p.m.

Use a lot of sunscreens and reapply every two hours, or more frequently if you're swimming or sweating.

Importance of this step: Your skin will turn red and inflamed when you get sunburned. As a result, any acne you already have will only get worse. Acne can get worse and even cause scarring from inflammation, which can be even more difficult to treat than acne. Additionally, sun exposure can make scarring and other dark spots stand out even more.

Sun exposure without sunscreen can also dry out and make your skin more oily, which can lead to acne. You might believe that the sun is beneficial to your skin. However, in reality, a nice tan only temporarily conceals acne. However, your acne will still be present when the tan wears off. In the long run, using sunscreen every day is better for your skin.

Right sunscreen for your skin: Using the right kind of sunscreen is very important if you get acne a lot. For acne-prone skin, sunscreen should be containing some ingredients like Niacinamide, Lactic acid, and Hyaluronic acid.

One of the best things you can do for your skin is to just follow these three steps and live a healthy life. If you choose your food well, get enough sleep, and drink a lot of water, these steps can be effective and healthy.

Some Other Tips For Healthy Skin

It is pretty understandable if you have no time for thorough skin care. You can still indulge yourself by mastering the fundamentals. Skin problems can be avoided and the natural aging process slowed down with good skincare and healthy lifestyle choices. Start with these straightforward suggestions.

Be Gentle With Your Skin

- Daily shaving and cleansing can be hard on your skin. To keep things light:

- Reduce the amount of time spent in the bathtub: Oils are removed from your skin by taking long baths or showers in hot water. Use warm water instead of hot water when taking a bath or shower.

- Use mild soaps instead: Detergents and strong soaps can strip oil from your skin. Choose mild cleaners instead.

- Shave with care: Before shaving, apply shaving cream, lotion, or gel to lubricate and protect your skin. Use a clean, sharp razor for the closest shave possible. Shave in the opposite direction of the hair's growth.

- Clean up: Use a towel to gently pat or blot your skin dry after a bath or shower to keep some moisture on your skin.

Avoid Smoking

Smoking contributes to wrinkles and makes your skin appear older. Smoking constricts the tiniest blood vessels in the skin's outermost layers, reducing blood flow and making the skin paler. Additionally, oxygen and nutrients essential to skin health are depleted as a result.

Collagen and elastin, the fibers that give your skin its strength and elasticity, are also damaged by smoking. When you smoke, you also make the same facial expressions over and over again, like squinting your eyes to keep smoke out and pursing your lips as you inhale.

Also, smoking makes you more likely to get squamous cell skin cancer. If you smoke, quitting is the best way to protect your skin. You can get help quitting smoking from your doctor.

Get Enough Sleep

Your cellular tissues are repaired and restored during your body's shutdown, ensuring their optimal vitality. Not only is getting enough sleep good for your skin, but it can also help your heart, weight, mind, and more.

The five scientific explanations for how skin is affected by sleep are as follows:

➢ At night, the skin repairs itself: Preventing wrinkles and sagging caused by premature aging is made easier by maintaining firm, plump skin. Melatonin, a hormone produced during sleep, fights wrinkles, fine lines, and even skin cancer by acting as an antioxidant. One of the best skin benefits of getting enough sleep is that it may be the closest thing to the fountain of youth.

➢ Sleep deprivation weakens your immune system: Sleep deprivation affects how well the immune system works. The effects of not getting enough sleep on the skin should be especially taken into consideration by those with cystic acne; An infection of the P. acnes bacteria deep within the pores causes deep acne lesions, which are harder to treat when immunity is low. Sleeping well can make you more resistant to colds and viruses and improve your skin's health by lowering inflammation.

➢ Sleep and skin also benefit from hydration: Your skin will appear and feel more dry and dehydrated the less you sleep. Dehydration caused by lack of sleep is obvious on the skin: eyes that are sunken and swollen; dark spots; flaking; a complexion that is drab and pale. You may appear and feel off your game as well as sluggish and irritable if you don't drink enough water. *BioClarity Hydrating Masque* will give your cells a plump, hydrating appearance. There are a lot of energizing nutrients, cleansing clays, and beautiful fruits and herbs in this masque.

Have Plenty Of Water

Every cell in your body is hydrated through the blood when you drink enough water. Drinking more water helps lower blood sugar levels. Acne on the skin has been linked to a higher blood sugar level and a higher sugar intake. As a result, maintaining a healthy blood sugar level by drinking enough water, which also aids in skin detoxification, is essential.

Drinking plenty of water benefits in so many ways like:

➢ **Improves Skin Tone:** When you drink enough water, your body flushes out toxins and your skin gets healthier. Two cups of water, according to studies, can increase blood flow to the skin, giving it an even tone.

➢ **Decreases puffiness:** Your skin is actually retaining water to keep you hydrated when it appears puffy. When you don't drink enough water, this happens. Your face will look less puffy and less swollen if you drink enough water.

➤ **No more irritated skin on the face:** Lack of moisture can even cause dry flakes to form and crack. Your skin will not become sufficiently dry to itch if you drink enough water.

➤ **Skin that is tighter:** When you suddenly lose weight, your skin may start to sag. Drinking water, which restores the skin's elasticity, is helpful for both preventing sagging and tightening the skin in areas where it is most noticeable, like the upper arms, thighs, waistline, and jawline.

Detox For Acne Skin

We are, without a doubt, product addicts, but when it comes to acne, we prefer to take a more holistic approach rather than hoard spot treatments and cleansers. Addressing the issue internally reduces stress on the skin (and the body as a whole), especially for those of us who experience the drying and burning effects of acne treatments.

So, when we found out that spearmint tea is bad for acne, we decided to look into other ways to drink our way to a clearer complexion without using skincare products. More on this in the future. Since tea is the "Magic Eraser" of pimples, there are a lot of teas to choose from, but we've also included a few other tasty drinks to quench your thirst—for a smoother complexion.

1 - Turmeric Tea

Turmeric Tea Curcumin, a component of the spice turmeric, is well-known for its anti-inflammatory, antiviral, antioxidant, and antifungal properties. In the country Ayurveda, it is used to treat a variety of internal and external ailments. While turmeric is currently a popular ingredient for homemade masks, it can also be used to treat acne in the same way as tea by adding one teaspoon to hot water.

How to make it?

Step 1: Take 1 tsp of turmeric tea.

Step 2: Add hot water.

Step 3: Add half tsp honey(optional). Bless your skin with this magic drink.

2 - Kefir

Because the health of your skin is a lot like the health of your gut, taking probiotics from kefir is good for fighting off bad bacteria and reducing inflammation. Kefir has a stronger ability to fight acne thanks to the protein lactoferrin. In one study, participants who consumed 200 milligrams of lactoferrin-fermented fermented milk daily experienced a 12-week decrease in inflammatory acne lesions of almost 39%.

How to make it?

Step 1: In the jar, add 12 teaspoons of kefir grains.

Step 2: If you're using a jar with a clip top, add a pint of milk, leaving at least 5 cm of head room.

Step 3: Ferment for 18 to 24 hours on the worktop.

Step 4: In your jug or bottle, strain the kefir through the sieve or straining funnel. The grains are quite sturdy and can be stirred gently. Enjoy!

3 - Matcha Tea

A fad drink is packed with antioxidants, including epigallocatechin gallate (EGCG), which counteract the oxidation of sebum that occurs prior to acne formation. Consuming antioxidants also help to reduce signs of inflammation from the inside out. Because Matcha contains 137 times as many antioxidants as regular green tea, you can be sure that each cup provides a significant dose.

How to make it?

Step 1: Using a small sifter, sift 1-2 teaspoons of matcha into a cup.

Step 2: Add 2 oz. of hot water. Use barely boiling water for the best results.

Step 3: Whisk vigorously in a zigzag pattern until the tea resembles whipped cream.

Step 4 : Take advantage of your matcha tea right out of the bowl.

4 - Organic Tart Cherry Juice

Instead of reaching for the sugar-laden cherry juice cocktail from the grocery store, sip the real thing to reap its full skin benefits. Although tart cherry juice may be unpleasant to the palate, it is rich in antioxidants as well as vitamins A, B, C, and D, and it contributes to the pH balance of your skin. It is also anti-inflammatory and contains melatonin, which aids in sleep.

How to make it?

Step 1: Preheat the oven to 375 degrees F. Then in a medium-sized bowl, mix sugar, orange juice, cornstarch, and vanilla extract.

Step 2: Pour mixture over cherries and stir until well coated.

Step 3: Pour cherries into a 9-inch pie dish or an 8x8 baking dish.

Step 4: Bake for 45 minutes to 1 hour, or until the juices are bubbly and the cherries are soft.

Step 5: Serve warm or cold, with a dollop of whipped cream or ice cream if desired. Enjoy!

5 - Spearmint Tea

We here inform you that drinking two cups of organic spearmint tea every day reduces inflammatory acne lesions by 25% after one month and by 51% after three months—which is even more effective than using prescription medications. Amazing, isn't it? I tried it for myself, and the results were impressive (glowing skin, significantly fewer pimples, and less redness).

How to make it?

Step 1: Bring water to a boil in a pan.

Step 2; Turn off the heat. Leave for five minutes after adding the spearmint leaves.

Step 3: Tea should be strained into a mug or cup before drinking.

In conclusion, these are five great drinks that can help you get rid of acne and improve your skin's health. Organic tart cherry juice, spearmint tea, turmeric tea, Matcha tea, and kefir are all excellent options for reducing inflammation and bad bacteria. Add one or more of these drinks to your daily routine if you want to improve your skin's health in a more comprehensive way. It will be well worth it for your skin!

CONCLUSION

As we have seen, there are a number of ingredients that can be beneficial for acne-prone skin. These include tea tree oil, salicylic acid, and azelaic acid. Each of these ingredients has unique properties that can help to reduce the appearance of acne and improve the overall health of the skin.

The science and approach to managing acne have come a long way in recent years. We now know that acne is not caused by dirt or poor hygiene, but is instead the result of a complex interplay between hormones, bacteria, and inflammation. However, by having the know-how of what ingredients can help or aggravate your skin condition, the management of acne can be much easier.

The ingredients as we have seen are not just limited to topical solutions, but also include food items such as green tea, which can help to reduce inflammation from the inside out. So, make sure to include these ingredients in your daily skincare routine or diet to see the best results for acne-prone skin.

In the end, I'd like to recommend being on the lookout for new research and developments in the field of acne management as well as ingredients. As we have seen, there are always new and innovative ways to help improve the appearance of acne-prone skin.

Thank you for taking the time to read this guide on acne ingredients. I hope that it was informative and helpful in finding the right ingredients for skincare routines and acne management.

REFERENCES

Oge'. (2019). Acne Vulgaris: Diagnosis and Treatment. *American Family Physician, 100*(8). https://pubmed.ncbi.nlm.nih.gov/31613567/

Sutaria, A. H., Masood, S., & Schlessinger, J. (2022, May 8). *Acne Vulgaris.* Nih.gov; StatPearls Publishing. https://www.ncbi.nlm.nih.gov/books/NBK459173/

Eichenfield, D. Z., Sprague, J., & Eichenfield, L. F. (2021). Management of Acne Vulgaris. *JAMA, 326*(20), 2055. https://doi.org/10.1001/jama.2021.17633

Williams, H. C., Dellavalle, R. P., & Garner, S. (2012). Acne vulgaris. *The Lancet, 379*(9813), 361–372. https://doi.org/10.1016/s0140-6736(11)60321-8

Kraft, J., & Freiman, A. (2011). Management of acne. *Canadian Medical Association Journal, 183*(7), E430–E435. https://doi.org/10.1503/cmaj.090374

Tan, A. U., Schlosser, B. J., & Paller, A. S. (2018). A review of diagnosis and treatment of acne in adult female patients. *International Journal of Women's Dermatology, 4*(2), 56–71. https://doi.org/10.1016/j.ijwd.2017.10.006

Titus S;Hodge J. (2012). Diagnosis and treatment of acne. *American Family Physician*, 86(8). https://pubmed.ncbi.nlm.nih.gov/23062156/

Kurokawa, I., & Nakase, K. (2020). Recent advances in understanding and managing acne. *F1000Research*, 9, 792. https://doi.org/10.12688/f1000research.25588.1

Ayer, J. (2006). Acne: more than skin deep. *Postgraduate Medical Journal*, 82(970), 500–506. https://doi.org/10.1136/pgmj.2006.045377